The
PROSTATE
MIRACLE

The
PROSTATE
MIRACLE

New Natural Therapies That Can Save Your Life

Jesse A. Stoff, M.D.
and
Dallas Clouatre, Ph.D.

KENSINGTON BOOKS
www.kensingtonbooks.com

This book is not intended as a substitute for medical advice of physicians and should be used only in conjunction with the advice of your personal doctor. The reader should regularly consult a physician in matters relating to his health and particularly with respect to any symptoms that may require diagnosis or medical attention.

This book is focused on treating prostate cancer, a potentially life-threatening disease and not appropriate for self-treatment.

KENSINGTON BOOKS are published by

Kensington Publishing Corp.
850 Third Avenue
New York, NY 10022

Copyright © 2000 by Jesse A. Stoff, M.D. and Dallas Clouatre, Ph.D.

ISBN 1-57566-544-1

First Kensington Trade Paperback Printing: September, 2000
10 9 8 7 6 5 4

Printed in the United States of America

Every success Dr. Stoff achieves significantly eases suffering and advances his very clear vision of a medical treatment modality that would succeed by benefiting everyone. The world needs to listen carefully. The possibilities offered by this approach to medical treatment cannot be equaled by any other ideas that my colleagues or I have encountered elsewhere.

—David L. Bergsma
President, Quantum Research, Inc.
Scottsdale, Arizona

An inspired book that (successfully) challenges the conventional oncology paradigms of today and offers realistic hope for those with prostate cancer . . . leads the way for enlightened oncology care in the new millennium.

—Dr. Yulius Poplyansky
Director of the International Foundation
for Innovative Medicine

To my gentle wife, Colleen, for without her unconditional love, support, and understanding, this book would not have been possible.

To my three wonderful children—Laurel, Spencer, and Summer—who delight, challenge, and sometimes frustrate me but whose presence is always a welcome gift from God.

To my father, Sheldon P. Stoff, who taught me the importance of balancing intellect with intuition, thus giving me new eyes with which to see.

To my mother, Lorraine Marshak Stoff, who through her patient love taught me to see beauty in the world, thus giving me the strength to be compassionate with those I meet.

To my brother, Josh, who by tenaciously pursuing his own dreams showed me that it was possible for me to fulfill mine.

To my mentors, Dr. George Olson, Dr. Bernie Siegel, Dr. Ben Papermaster, Bears Kaufman, and Dr. Jim B. Peter, scholars and gentlemen all, who have graciously given me broad shoulders to stand upon that I may see a bit further.

To Claire Gerus, assistant Richard Ember, and to editor and patient Lee Heiman, who was diagnosed with prostate cancer while we were writing this book, and then courageously embarked upon a healing journey of his own for the first time in his life.

Jesse A. Stoff, M.D.
Tucson, Arizona, 2000

Do not pray for an easy life;
pray for greater strength.
Do not pray for tasks equal to your powers;
pray for powers equal to your tasks.
Then the doing of your work shall be no miracle;
but you will be a miracle.
Every day you will wonder at yourself;
at the richness of the life that has come to you
by the grace of God.
Faith is walking to the edge of all you have . . .
and taking one more step.

—Anonymous

Statement from Walter Zacharius
Chairman of the Board, Kensington Publishing

Lee Heiman, one of our health editors, has chosen to describe his own experience with prostate cancer in this book. In so doing, he has offered us intimate access to the personal side of this disease—a courageous undertaking, but not surprising to those of us who know Lee and his tireless dedication to the cause of health.

Lee willingly made himself a test subject of Dr. Jesse Stoff's program because he trusted that it could help him heal his cancer. He tells me that his trust was well placed, and that he continues to improve daily.

Lee's story will both inspire and support any man facing the prospect of this disease. It will also help all of us who seek insights and hope for our own personal journeys on the road to wellness.

CONTENTS

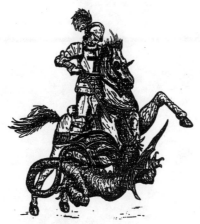

Drawing by Josh Stoff

One of the most ancient archetypes is the image of the sword. Countless other weapons have come and gone but even today, in the age of missiles and nuclear fission, the image of the sword is more than a weapon against foes of flesh and blood. It symbolizes willpower, the power which, if used correctly, can conquer the evil existing as a possibility in all men.

Its slender, radiant blade is an image of the rays of the sun, bringing light into darkness. With its point turned downward, it has always been a symbol of peace. It is not by accident that its hilt is shaped like a cross.

Thus, since time immemorial, the hero's sword appears in legends and myths as an image of creative will, its blade of light subduing the dragon on earth. If man wants to be free and to subdue the dragon in himself, he must learn to wield a sacred sword.

—*Dr. Franz Winkler*

FOREWORD

One out of three American men can expect to develop cancer in his lifetime. The good news is that Dr. Jesse Stoff has created a clinically proven and extremely logical eclectic blend of allopathic, naturopathic, and nutritional medicine that has brought hope and remissions to hundreds of his cancer patients. After 18 years of clinical practice, most of Dr. Stoff's prostate cancer patients are still alive. This is good news, indeed, for the readers of this book and users of the Stoff approach to the diagnosis and treatment of cancer.

Cancer is a whole body disease, not just a regional lump or bump. Therefore, cancer requires whole body therapies, not merely isolated and highly toxic stabs at the blatant problem areas. The simplistic model of Western medicine and research isolates one variable. But that's not the way that the body works. The human body is an elegant spiritual machine, composed of 60 trillion interdependent and synergistic cells that create an amazingly complex yet wondrous human life. The simplistic model of medicine states: "If you can name it, then I can tame it." Yet, that same reigning medical system has failed to prevent or reverse many common degenerative diseases among Americans, including many forms of cancer, heart disease, hypertension, diabetes, arthritis, immune disorders like multiple sclerosis, osteoporosis, and an assortment of mental disorders.

The groundbreaking approach that Dr. Stoff has developed for treating cancer patients pays homage to the complexity of the human body and recognizes that no two cancer patients are alike, either in the underlying causes of the disease or in therapeutic treatment. No one with a headache is suffering from a deficiency of aspirin. And no one with prostate cancer has a deficiency of Lupron™, radiation therapy, or surgery. The Stoff protocol of treatment gets to the root of the problem. Once the underlying cause of the disease has been identified and reversed, the prostate cancer patient stands a good chance of going into remission or at least finding dramatic improvement in quality and quantity of life.

As we enter a new millennium, it is very reassuring to me to find Jesse Stoff, M.D., leading the way toward a new healing system that is more clinically effective, more humane, and more cost effective. Ignaz Semmelweiss was a nineteenth-century Austrian physician who found that washing hands before delivering a baby could dramatically cut the incidence of maternal infections after childbirth. His ideas were scorned then, but make perfectly good sense now. I put Dr. Stoff in the same category of brilliance, altruism, and determination. It is your good fortune to have this book in your hands. Best wishes for a speedy recovery from your prostate cancer.

—Patrick Quillin, Ph.D., R.D., C.N.S., and author
Vice President of Nutrition
Cancer Treatment Centers of America

Introduction

One day everything is going along fine as usual. The next day, you have a doctor's appointment and suddenly your world is turned upside down. You have prostate cancer. Shock, fear, questions—lots of questions. How long, how bad, is it going to hurt? What do I do now? I want help, I want the best, I want to know, I want to have, to share, to do so much. I want to live!

Few of us react well to a diagnosis of cancer. I write this based upon long experience, for cancer has been a scourge in my family. As a little boy, I lost two grandmothers and an aunt to breast cancer. There was no help for them. When I asked my mother what cancer was, she hesitated a moment and then said, "You're too young to worry about it." Twenty years later she, too, was stricken with breast cancer.

Perhaps as a result, my childhood dream was to become a doctor. Our family physician was a homeopathic practitioner, and my early experiences in medicine were in the form of homeopathy. In fact, while I was in high school, I accompanied my family doctor/friend to homeopathic conferences. Later, I studied homeopathy in London, followed by attendance at an allopathic medical school to become an M.D. This sequence of events may help to explain my willingness to try a variety of unconventional approaches to the treatment of cancer. It certainly helped to prepare me for the next round of cancer in my own family.

When my mother was diagnosed with breast cancer, she was already at the advanced stage four level. The cancer was in her arm bones, skull, breastbone, and innumerable other places. Her oncologist, a prominent member of the profession, told her that with surgery, radiation, and chemotherapy she should "survive" another six months. With all of her strength and courage, Mom said no to his idea of "survival" and called me. Together we embarked upon a search for healing. Now, ten years later, she is still in clinical remission. Ever since I helped find relief for my mother's condition, I have sought to create a practice in which my patients could benefit from my approach to treating cancer.

"Help" is what this book is all about. Help with understanding your cancer. Help with information resources. Help with the latest protocols available in integrative oncology for prostate cancer that are working with my patients. Help for you to focus on the quality of your life.

If you have been diagnosed with prostate cancer, you have lots of company. Prostate cancer is the most common form of cancer in men. It also is roughly one-third more common in men than breast cancer is in women. Of course, most men do not give prostate cancer much thought unless they suddenly find themselves or a friend diagnosed with it—it is not a "high-profile" cancer, not the darling of media attention. Nor is prostate cancer a benign condition. It is very real, and many men do die from it—between 35,000 and 40,000 American men last year alone.

For most men, and certainly for most of my patients, prostate cancer is not an automatic sentence of death or disability. Of those individuals diagnosed today with prostate cancer, almost 90 percent will still be alive in five years and more than 60 percent will still be alive in ten years. These are not bad odds for a cancer in which 80 percent of the diagnosed cases are in men already 65 years of age or older!

Now there is even better news. If you already have prostate cancer, you *can* do something to positively affect your condition. Medical treatment options are broad and are becoming more so. New complementary therapies and integrative treatment protocols can have a powerful impact upon your rate of recovery from prostate cancer. You can take control of factors such as diet, supplements, exercise, therapies to reduce stress and its effect on your immune system, etc., to dramatically improve your chances of surviving prostate cancer, *and of surviving it with your quality of life intact!*

Some new treatments available for prostate cancer have gone a long way toward improving your chances of successfully surviving this condition while maintaining a normal life. One of these is the herbal treatment known as PC SPES. A recent flurry of positive medical trials has suddenly brought this "alternative" or "complementary" medical treatment to the attention of the world of orthodox cancer doctors. PC SPES appears to be especially useful for reducing prostate-specific antigen (PSA) scores and for improving the general clinical status of patients, i.e., patients tend to feel better and to experience improved quality of life. This book not only explains what PC SPES is and how it works, but also goes well beyond this to show you how to get the most benefits from a synergistic treatment program of immunotherapy in combination with PC SPES. *No other book available provides specific, clinically proven, integrated medical protocols designed to enhance your quality and quantity of life and therefore allow you to live many more fruitful years.*

The cornerstone of the approach I take in my practice, "integrative oncology," is a custom-tailored, individualized approach that recognizes the uniqueness of every individual who has cancer.

Cancer is not an arbitrary and random event, nor is it an automatic death sentence. It occurs when several complex and integrated biological systems fail, the cause of which is different in each case. What contributes to these failures? Family background, personal history, diet, exposure to environmental toxins, and lifestyle habits. Fortunately, specialized blood tests and a host of markers and guideposts can discover the weaknesses that lead to cancer and to uncover the strengths that can help you fight back.

This is the message of our book. You can experience prostate cancer as a challenge to be overcome. You *can* fight back and do so successfully! Within these pages are the tools to help you and your doctor meet this challenge, including information on the most promising immunological and holistic therapies, such as the herbal product PC SPES. Yet fundamentally our book is about hope, and our goal is to show you how to get well and be one of the victors!

Who Should Read This Book?

Several different audiences can benefit from this book. The obvious audience consists of men who have just been diagnosed with prostate cancer. These men usually are troubled by feelings of confusion and denial. All the classic questions come up, beginning with those about the nature of cancer itself and then turning to the issues of treatment options and the prognosis for the future.

Of course, not everyone waits until an actual personal diagnosis of prostate cancer to worry about this condition. Anyone with family or friends with a history of cancer, such as I have, will be sensitive to the topic. Each of us has our own little platoon of humanity whose cares and fears become, in some sense, our own.

African-American men in particular should be concerned with the information found on the following pages. For reasons that remain obscure, African-American men suffer from roughly twice the rate of diagnosis of and death from, prostate cancer as those in other populations. Moreover, black men are younger when they discover they have active prostate cancer, many even before age 50. In white men, such risk rates are typical only in those with a genetic propensity to prostate cancer as may be indicated by having brothers or a father who has developed this condition.

Any disease or medical condition affects not only the patient, but also his spouse and other family and friends. Therefore, the wife and family of prostate cancer patients will want to learn all they can about this condition and its treatment. Dietary changes, stress reduction, and other such complementary therapies can be extremely important to assist in recovery from prostate cancer. This means that the patient's immediate family cannot help but be involved. These therapies may have a substantial impact upon "normal" everyday habits. Knowing why these therapies are being undertaken and what to expect can go a long way toward making alterations in long-standing routines less difficult.

Finally, this book is intended for physicians, nutritionists, nurses, and other health care professionals involved with the treatment of prostate cancer. This field of oncology is undergoing a period of rapid change. Moreover, because men with prostate cancer increasingly are seeking to become better informed and to be more active in their own treatment programs, it is now more important for doctors to know what their patients are doing and why. Not all "complementary" therapies can be used with standard allopathic treatments. Little is gained if doctor and patient find themselves acting at crossed purposes.

What to Expect

Most men who contract prostate cancer can lead productive and fulfilling lives long *after* diagnosis. Therefore, if you have recently been diagnosed with prostate cancer, do not give your fears a head start.

Instead, your first order of business is to learn all you can about prostate cancer: its possible causes, and how to initiate the healing process.

You may be surprised to learn that cancerous tissues are just like other tissues, but less healthy. Like other tissues, cancerous tissues must be fed. And, like other tissues, cancerous tissues must arrange for the removal of wastes. Cancerous tissues must also reproduce, just like other tissues. They must also remain off the "attack radar" of the immune system.

The good news is, cancerous tissues are vulnerable. There are ways to cut off the food supply to cancerous tissues. There are ways to prevent cancerous tissues from efficiently getting rid of waste materials, thus retarding their growth. There are ways to inhibit the reproduction of cancerous cells, and to cause cancerous cells to program their own deaths. There are ways to make cancerous tissues once again "pop up" on the immune system's "radar." There are even ways to coax the cancer cells to return to normal.

The following chapters provide a road map to help you and your doctor to do just these things. Expect to learn all of the following and much more, including:

- What prostate cancer is, and whether there is a prostate cancer "epidemic."
- The suspected causes of prostate cancer.
- How prostate cancer is detected. When to get a second opinion.

- The fourfold treatment foundation and when to look for alternatives.
- Dietary intervention—the truth about fats, meat, caloric restrictions, vegetarian diets, and other options.
- Why detoxification is so important.
- Beyond PSA: Determining what the cancer is doing via specialized blood, tissue, and other tests.
- Gauging the strength of the immune system.
- Your biochemical individuality and how it affects your cancer.
- The right supplement for the right patient to do the right job.
- Understanding neuroimmunology: Why stress is your enemy and how emotions can cripple your endocrine and immune systems.
- Where to look for moral support.
- How to meet the challenge to change.

If you are curious whether your blood type matters in creating a treatment protocol, then read on. If you have heard of calcium-D-glucarate, coenzyme Q-10, genistein, lycopene shark liver oil, seleniums, plant sterols and sterolins, flower pollen extract, AIDECWE or a dozen other herbs and supplements and wonder whether they can help you in fighting against prostate cancer, this is the book for you.

How to Use This Book

Although fighting prostate cancer is definitely **not** a matter of "self-help" treatments—you'll need advice and treatment from a competent, sympathetic physician/oncologist—there are still many steps you can take yourself to speed your recovery:

- You can change your eating habits.
- You can get moderate daily exercise and adequate sunshine.
- You can find ways of relieving stress and anxiety.
- You can add appropriate supplements to your diet.

Part One of this book, "Understanding Prostate Cancer," offers an overview of the subject and gives you the vocabulary you'll need to understand "doctor speak." You will learn about the impressive results achieved with PC SPES and clinical immunology, as well as guidelines for a health-boosting diet and supplementation.

You will also find my personal suggestions for the steps you can take on your own. "Dr. Jesse's Tips" are helpful hints as to which foods to avoid, which to add, and why. The last chapter in this part describes one man's experience with prostate cancer and his discovery that lifestyle changes and treatment can offer far more hope than one might expect.

Part Two, "A Return to Balance," is for you and your physician. Always keep in mind that your doctor is your partner in your fight against prostate cancer. Don't be dismayed when you find that many or even most of the compounds suggested at the end of the later chapters are prescription items. Your doctor can get these for you, but he must understand why these various items are clinically useful. Let your doctor share this book with you—you'll both be glad that you did.

Part Three, "On the Road to Healing," provides an integrated approach to battling prostate cancer. Here, you will find an overview of your "plan of attack." Just as important, you will be reminded that your attitude can be a key ingredient in the fight against cancer. This battle involves more than just pills and potions. Success depends upon your spirit.

You'll find that I have supplied phone numbers and relevant information on prescription items, unusual blood tests, and the like in the Appendix. I also include lists of physicians' organizations. These are important sources of information for you in your quest for a physician who is sympathetic toward putting my protocols into practice. Physicians may check out protocols, dosages and labs in a special section in the Appendix.

Remember, your life is in your hands, as is the power to find the medical help that is best for you.

PART ONE

Understanding Prostate Cancer

CHAPTER ONE

Prostate Cancer and You

By reading this book and following its suggestions, with the support of your physician, you are taking the first steps on what may be the most challenging journey of your life. This journey will help you discover exactly how you can begin the healing process, and believe me, there is a *lot* you can do.

We will give you clinically proven information to answer the "where" and "how" to find the answers to your questions. But you will have to meet us halfway by opening your mind and your heart to accept our help. We'll then begin to journey the road less traveled together.

Newly diagnosed prostate cancer patients usually have the same questions. Providing the answers is a good way for us to begin our journey together.

1. What is cancer?
2. Am I alone, or is there a prostate cancer epidemic?
3. What are my chances of developing prostate cancer?
4. Could I have done something different, for instance, with my diet, to have prevented this?
5. What are my diagnostic and treatment options?
6. What about those prostate supplements you so often hear

about for enlarged prostates (saw palmetto, flower pollen extracts, whatever)? Will they work for me?

7. I've been told that there are some really advanced (or ancient?) therapies, like PC SPES—should I start with these and just skip more conventional treatments?

We'll discuss the last three questions in later chapters. The present chapter addresses the first four of these questions. As many a cancer survivor will tell you, it is never too late to adopt more healthful habits. Seemingly hopeless cases of cancer go into remission every day, and in most of these "miracles" one will find that the patient (often with the advice and encouragement of the attending physician) took active measures to turn around both his dietary and his emotional habits. Left to its own devices, and with the roadblocks to healing removed, the body will do what comes naturally to it—it heals!

Let's start with an overview of my understanding of prostate cancer. Patients with prostate cancer should try to develop their own

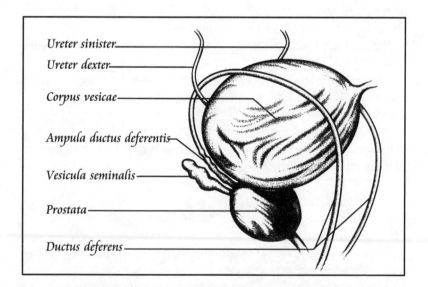

Figure 1. The Prostate Gland. The prostate lies under and slightly in front of the bladder, here called the *Corpus vesicae*. The ureters lead from the kidneys to the bladder. The *Ductus deferens* originate in the testes.

understanding of their condition. My approach to prostate cancer is different from that of many other doctors. I do not view cancer as being merely a cellular disturbance occurring in a specific organ or tissue. I do not believe that cancer occurs in isolation from activities in the rest of the body. I *do* believe that just as prostate cancer is preceded by related changes elsewhere in the body, so also does the treatment of prostate cancer require the treatment of the entire person, not just the prostate gland.

Remember, *cancer is a systemic disease*; it is the result of wide-ranging, fundamental changes in the body. In order for cancer to occur, multiple roadblocks to healing had to occur first. These include the failure of numerous biochemical and immunological systems due to infection, the buildup of toxins, or of one or more nutritional deficiencies. These prior changes neutralized the body's normal protection, which would have eliminated the cancerous cells before they had a chance to reproduce. Defeating cancer requires addressing the initial infection(s), toxin(s) or deficiencies responsible for the underlying bodily weakness. It also means aligning all your physical, mental, and spiritual resources to create *a united movement toward health*.

Therapies that target the cancer tissue itself, such as radiation, surgery, and chemotherapy, may be life-prolonging, but do nothing to address the underlying abnormalities that allowed the disease to manifest. Therefore, the therapeutic approach I take is not one of just treating the cancer (I'm not an oncologist). Instead, as an immunologist, I work with organs and systems of the body to improve their functioning. This includes helping the body rid itself of the toxins that may have triggered and/or accelerated the cancer cells' growth. The therapies I offer are as comprehensive as is necessary to address the multiple underlying dysfunctions.

In my practice, I use laboratory testing at the best reference labs available in the United States to identify each patient's biochemical and immunological abnormalities. (Several reference laboratories will be identified in later chapters.) I'll then recommend therapy with nutritional supplements to address the abnormalities and deficiencies identified, thus laying a foundation for the immune system to regain its strength. Based upon the individual's health situation and the latest medical research, I'll use the best natural medicines from all over the world to help rebuild the immune system. I'll also recommend acupuncture and homeopathy to reenergize the functioning of the immune system. I'll share with you other therapies to detoxify your body and ease stress on your mental, emotional, and spiritual levels. This comprehensive holistic approach is designed to coax the body's organs and systems in the direction of health and to bring about the best possible prognosis. I'll also recommend physicians who will support you in working with the treatments I discuss throughout this book (see the Appendix).

What Is Cancer?

Medical textbooks will tell you that there are hundreds of types of cancer, but the common thread is that cancer cells are abnormal and multiply at accelerated rates. Whereas normal cells play specific roles in the body and their growth is closely regulated by various signals, cancer cells seemingly exist primarily to reproduce. These wild cells expand beyond their local origin to invade adjacent tissues. Often, in a process called *metastasis*, stray cells will break free into the bloodstream and implant themselves in other parts of the body distant from the original site. This propensity to invade surrounding tissues and to metastasize separates cancers, or *malignancies,* from benign tumors, such as warts and polyps.

Our bodies' organ system is made up of different tissues, which, in turn, are made up of a variety of cells. Not all of these cells are dividing at any one time. Instead, the functions and replication rates of the cells are closely regulated by cellular DNA (deoxyribonucleic acid), the genetic "blueprint" of the cells found inside each nucleus. The DNA strands themselves consist of genes, the individual packets of instructions to the cells. Chemical signals, usually in the form of small protein molecules, constantly enter each cell from the bloodstream and interact with the mechanisms that control which genes will be active and which will not. Similarly, microscopic tubules are beneath the structure of the cell and extend outside of it to touch neighboring cells. These tubules, too, are part of the body's communications network. Cancer cells have in some fashion either ceased to respond to the body's communications and regulatory networks, or are responding in a way that is hazardous to the order and survival of the whole.

One way of looking at cancer cells is to view them as "permanently juvenile" cells that never "grow up." Mature normal cells are said to be "differentiated," which means that they have taken on shapes and characteristics that make them specific to their particular functions in the body, and different from other cells. Cancer cells might be said to have had their development arrested at a stage prior to full differentiation.

This way of looking at cancer cells is important in treatment because cancer cells that are forced to differentiate are less virulent, less damaging, and act more like normal cells. As will be shown in later chapters, it is sometimes possible through the use of certain nutrients to *return cancer cells to normal* or near normal structure and behavior. I employ nutritional treatment routinely when dealing with prostate cancer because such protocols are necessary for success.

Even normal, or "good" cells can go "bad." For example, the genes that normally provide the instructions for the process of replication (*proto-oncogenes*) may become damaged in some fashion. When this happens, the resulting *oncogene* becomes like a switch that has been left in the "on" position, when it should have been turned off. Therefore, the cell begins to replicate uncontrollably. In the new cells into which the cell divides, the oncogene is now the pattern for replication, and cell division is no longer properly linked to the cell's tissue function, needs, or signals from the body as a whole.

The proto-oncogenes of normal cells are themselves regulated or controlled by *tumor suppressor genes*, which usually serve as "watchdogs" to make sure that the cell is acting as it should. There are, in fact, two identical sets of tumor suppressor genes in each cell. If one set fails, the other set will still be able to oversee cellular operations. These genes are, in effect, the master set that rule how the other instructions (genes) that make up the cellular DNA are to be read and acted upon. If both sets somehow become damaged, the cell will cease to behave like a normal cell of its kind, may radically change its shape, and may begin to replicate itself without any control.

The body has a variety of mechanisms to protect itself against unwanted changes in the DNA, as the genes are the basic code to regulate all bodily processes. One of the most important of these mechanisms, which is lately becoming increasingly appreciated by scientists, is called *methylation*. Methyl groups are single carbon units with the structure CH_3 (one carbon and three hydrogen atoms). Methylation refers to the attachment of one or more methyl groups to different substances. This process has an impact upon the body that starts at the most elementary level—how DNA is expressed in the genes.

Methyl groups are attached at special sites to the DNA to protect against the expression or activation of genes that can cause many diseases, including cancer. Indeed, almost all cancers, not just prostate cancer, become much more common in later life due to our declining ability to replace the methyl groups located on the DNA strands as we grow older. Fortunately, as you will be discover, it is possible to improve the body's supply of methyl groups by eating certain foods, such as beets, and taking particular supplements—all of which we will talk about later.

Kinds of Cancer

Cancers are classified according to the type of tissue from which they originated. The four major types of cancer are *leukemia, lymphoma, sarcoma, and carcinoma*. Leukemia is cancer of the blood cells and typically begins in the bone marrow, where new blood cells are formed. Lymphoma, as name suggests, arises in the tissues of the lymphatic system, such as the lymph nodes. Sarcoma develops in bone or connective tissues.

Prostate cancer is a form of carcinoma, as are the preponderance of all cancers, including lung, breast, colon, and skin cancers. These cancers all develop into solid tumors and arise from epithelial tissues, which cover the surface of the body (i.e., the skin) as well as line all the internal cavities of the body.

Unfortunately, both patients and their doctors tend to think of cancer as a largely autonomous growth that no longer fits into the body's regulatory, signaling, and communications networks. Yet, it has long been known that surgery on the primary site of a cancer will affect the rate of growth and other aspects of metastasized portions of the cancer found in distant parts of the body. It can slow down or speed up the growth of cancerous tissues elsewhere in the body. However, it is still not clear whether surgery will affect other cancerous areas positively or negatively.

Cancerous cells are, in fact, responding to at least some of the signals being sent out by the organism as a whole. Even the description of the dysfunctional oncogenes and failed tumor suppressor genes just a few paragraphs earlier largely assumes that these alterations are not responding to actual signals being sent by the system as a whole, or that the development of the cancer is a response to an abnormal internal environment.

In a famous article published in *Science* in 1956, researcher Otto Warburg argued that cancer cells originate as a long-term response to failures in energy production within tissues. By this he meant that cancer cells in animals act less and less like true animal cells and more like plant or yeast cells. The changes include becoming less dependent upon oxygen and more likely to produce energy in an oxygen-poor environment than is true of normal cells. Some aspects of this line of argument have been revived by a number of our contemporary cancer specialists.

Very curiously, cancer very seldom develops in contractile tissues, that is, in muscle tissues. One can, of course, perhaps give all sorts of chemical and genetic explanations for this exception. However, it is very tempting to wonder whether this is because muscle tissues can contract to release tension and stress. We know that the so-called Type A personality—the driven and anger-prone personality—manifests elevated rates of heart disease. There are other personality types that are also associated with elevated rates of cancer. Statistically speaking, the prostate cancer personality seems to be one of inward-turning stress, as opposed to the outward-turning anger and action of the Type A personality.

The emotions and "fuzzy" factors such as purpose, fulfillment, and peace of mind can powerfully affect the immune and endocrine systems. Both of these systems are intimately linked to the development of cancer. The endocrine system releases hormones that can spur on, or deactivate, tumor growth.

Am I Alone, Or Is There a PC Epidemic?

The truth is, most men ignore their prostate gland until something goes wrong with it. Unfortunately, over the last decade, several celebrities have found themselves admitting quite publicly that something has gone wrong with this inconspicuous little gland. Former senator Bob Dole, author Michael Korda, and retired General Norman Schwarzkopf readily come to mind. But these men are not alone. Why have the prostate and its problems suddenly become so public?

The short answer is that, according to figures from the American Cancer Society and other authorities, the number of diagnosed cases of prostate cancer increased from roughly 85,000 in 1985 to some 99,000 in 1988, and then to between 200,000 to more than 317,000 in 1996. This is an increase of 200 to 300 percent in a mere ten years! One leading cancer specialist, Curtin Mettlin, M.D., of the Roswell Park Cancer Institute of New York, says that the rise in prostate cancer represents the most dramatic upward change in the incidence of a specific disease in this century.

Does this mean there's an epidemic of prostate cancer in the United States at the beginning of the twenty-first century? Many doctors would answer this question with a resounding "No!" Others would point out that the rise in prostate cancer is in line with increases in other cancers. Moreover, even those authorities who deny that there is an epidemic of prostate cancer are split on whether new diagnostic methods and earlier detection actually improve the quality of life of their cancer patients.

How, you might ask, can a 300 percent jump in ten years *not* constitute an epidemic? Well, the main reason these figures may be misleading is that detection techniques have improved. The prostate-specific antigen (PSA) test was first approved for general use in 1985. This analytic procedure is much more sensitive than the older digital rectal exam (DRE), which depends upon the doctor being able to feel changes in the prostate gland. In addition, before symptoms appear, prostate cancer must have grown to a significant degree. Yet it only takes a relatively small number of cancer cells to cause a rise in PSA scores. Therefore, the number of newly diagnosed prostate cancer cases could have risen merely because of the better detection afforded by the PSA test.

Such an improvement in early detection does not automatically mean that men's health is improved by early diagnosis. It is now known that perhaps 40 percent of all men between the ages of 30 and 50 have precancerous prostate lesions. Yet most cases of clinically active prostate cancer are found only in men aged 65 and above. Unlike breast cancer, which can double in size in three months, about 50 percent of all diagnosed prostate cancers require five years to double in size. This means that prostate cancer is usually among the slowest-growing of all cancers. Some doctors believe that many of the older men who currently are being diagnosed with prostate cancer are at very early stages of development. If not for the new techniques, they would have lived out their lives without ever knowing they had cancer. Only 19 percent of all prostate cancer deaths occur before the age of 70, and approximately 42 percent of all prostate cancer-related deaths occur after the age of 80. At these advanced ages, competing causes of death are very common. Therefore the prevention of death from prostate cancer will not necessarily prolong life.

The downside to this "ignorance-is-bliss" argument is that early detection in men *not* already in advanced old age allows for proper treatment and changes in living habits. These could save at least some of those 35,000 to 40,000 men who die of prostate cancer each year. In fact, prostate cancer is the most common cause of cancer deaths in men over the age of 50.

What Are My Chances of Developing It?

It would be nice to be able to conclude that there is no dramatic increase in the incidence of prostate cancer. Unfortunately, we have no data that can tell us absolutely that the increased rate of diagnosis is simply due to improved detection methods. Moreover, there are quite good reasons for suspecting that something other than a better detection methodology is at work. For instance, the rate of testicular cancer, normally found in men under 35 years of age, has increased sharply in recent decades. Similarly, sperm counts have fallen by about one-half over the last 50 years, and the relative rate of decline in sperm counts is higher in today's younger men than in those of the previous generation. One suspected cause of these cancers and sperm declines is the various synthetic estrogens (xenoestrogens) now found in our environment. For instance, not only pesticides and herbicides, but even many common plastics and household chemicals, can be absorbed by our bodies and can actually send out estrogen-like hormonal growth signals to our cells. Personally, I am very cautious about both the food and the environment to which I expose my children, my wife, and myself.

Genetics also plays a role in determining which men will develop prostate cancer. Certainly African-American men are more at risk both for developing prostate cancer, and for developing it at an earlier age. Today, the overall risk of developing prostate cancer is about 40 percent higher in black males than in white males. Because highly pigmented skin reduces the body's ability to synthesize vitamin D, and lower relative blood levels of vitamin D have been linked to the development of prostate cancer, researchers believe that the higher rate of prostate cancer in black men is related to this factor. Of course, other factors may also be involved.

More significant for prostate cancer than racial type in terms of genetics is the family history. The risk of developing prostate cancer is twice as high in those men who have one other member of their immediate family (father or brother) who developed the cancer. If two other members of the immediate family have developed the cancer, then the risk is fivefold. This would suggest that those who have prostate cancer in the family should adopt appropriate dietary and other health habits as a precaution. The old saying about "an ounce of prevention" is always good advice when it comes to cancer.

The Enemies Within

Cancer does not just pop up out of the blue. Most researchers accept that there is a sequence of stages, or events, leading to the appearance of a true cancer.

In the first step, either a *procarcinogen* or a *carcinogen* leads to the *initiation* of the cancer. That is, it causes the initial genetic damage. A carcinogen directly initiates the development of the cancer, whereas a procarcinogen requires the action of an activating enzyme from the body before it can initiate cancerous changes. An example of how activating enzymes work is given below in the discussion of liver enzymes. After initiation, the process must pass through the stages of *promotion* (such as through the impact of chronic inflammation or infection) and *progression* before the *cancer* develops. The next stage is *metastasis*, the spread of the cancer to tissues beyond the original site. Therefore, the stages of cancer development are initiation, promotion, progression, cancer, and metastasis.

Quite a number of factors have been suggested as causes of cancer in general, and prostate cancer in particular. These factors can be broadly divided into those involving oxidation and free radicals, and those involving the failure of the body to detoxify itself.

There are also suggestions that the levels of hormones and other compounds natural to our bodies can be too elevated or can otherwise initiate cancer. Once these ways of looking at procarcinogens and carcinogens have been explained, more specific elements can be examined. For instance, if one believes that a high-fat diet causes prostate cancer, one must still decide whether this is because fats generate more free radicals, or because they inhibit the detoxification pathways, or because fats cause dysregulation of hormone levels. Therefore, it is worthwhile to begin with the general theories before getting down to specifics.

By far, the most widely known factor suggested as a cause of cancer is the action of free radicals. The "free radical" theory observes that oxygen appears everywhere in bodily reactions. *Glycolysis,* the cleaving of carbon bonds from carbohydrate molecules to release energy, creates free radicals. The burning of fats in anaerobic respiration (cellular energy produced without adequate oxygen) creates free radicals. The functioning of the immune system when large white blood cells attack invaders creates more free radicals. The mere presence of many minerals in the body, especially but not limited to iron and copper, provides catalysts that create free radicals. (I frequently measure my patients' metal levels so I can recommend the best ratios to fight free radicals.) The immune system's inflammation response, and the most primitive of our immune responses, also creates free radicals.

All these free radicals are simply atoms and molecules that carry one single electron. In chemistry, the term "radical" refers to a component that can be involved in many reactions in sequence without itself undergoing change. Free radicals typically initiate cascades of free radical formation, with each step creating yet another damaging radical. These radicals attack fats and proteins, damage cell membranes, inactivate important cell enzymes, and ultimately interfere with the cellular DNA strands. The methylation process mentioned earlier is one way the body protects its DNA against damage by free radicals.

Knocking Out Free Radicals

Free radicals can be scavenged or "put out of action" in many different ways. The simplest procedure is for an antioxidant to donate an electron—it is this electron that puts the free radical out of action—and then itself forms a stable molecule. Antioxidants are, by definition, substances that are very easily oxidized and which, when oxidized, become harmless and easily excretable or actually benefit the body. Vitamin C is perhaps the best-known example of these compounds.

Many scavenging processes require several steps. For instance, one type of radical known as the superoxide molecule (O_2^-) first is turned into the less reactive hydrogen peroxide (H_2O_2) by the enzyme superoxide dismutase (SOD), and then this hydrogen peroxide is converted to water and plain oxygen by glutathione. Glutathione, in turn, is made more effective in its role in the presence of vitamin C, which can be oxidized and then excreted. *Of particular interest with regard to prostate cancer: it is those prostate cells that are glutathione deficient that become cancerous.*

Lycopene, the bright red compound found in tomatoes and made more available to the body when tomatoes are cooked with a fat or oil, recently has been widely publicized as a reason that Italian men have relatively low levels of prostate cancer. Lycopene is a powerful antioxidant that is very friendly to the tissues of the prostate.

Antioxidants can block the initiation phase of cancer development, and usually the phases of promotion and progression as well. Once there is a full-blown cancer, however, things become a lot more complicated.

Because antioxidants cannot protect you against all of the forms of toxic assault, the body has other forms of protection available. Free radicals often initiate cancerous changes in cells, but not all carcinogens are free radicals. In fact, most potential cancer-causing compounds are *not* free radicals and only develop their ability to wreak havoc upon cellular DNA *after* the body has acted upon them.

In activating these procarcinogens, our own detoxification systems can be at fault. The liver—our chief detoxifying organ—uses a two-step enzymatic procedure to remove the bulk of toxins from the body, and both of these steps must work perfectly to properly eliminate poisonous compounds. Important support for these actions by the liver comes from supplements such as calcium D-glucarate and indole-3-carbinol, methyl donors—including S-adenosyl-methionine (SAMe) and trimethylglycine (TMG)—and enzyme building blocks such as N-acetyl-cysteine (NAC). These compounds play roles in the Phase I and Phase II enzyme detoxification pathways.

Detoxification

In Phase I of the liver's detoxification process, certain enzymes make fat-soluble toxins more water-soluble, preventing toxic compounds from being stored in fatty tissues and making it easier for them to be excreted from the body. The 50 to 100 enzymes involved in the Phase I system prepare potential carcinogens for elimination by the Phase II system. In a process known as "conjugation," the Phase II system uses enzymes to bind directly to the compounds that have been changed in Phase I, thus inactivating them. These conjugated (bound) toxins are then excreted. Most of the environmental toxins we encounter are fat-soluble compounds with hormonal actions (such as estrogen-like compounds in our air and food), and these must be eliminated through the actions of the Phase

I enzymes. (See Chapter 6, the section entitled "Surviving in a Toxic World.")

Unfortunately, Phase I system enzymes sometimes make poisonous compounds even more active as carcinogens until these compounds are fully conjugated. Water-soluble toxins, for instance, are more effective at gaining access to the DNA genetic element of the cells. Therefore, to protect against the initiation of cancers, the Phase II enzymes, which are directly involved in the excretion of toxins from the system, must always be working as actively as are the Phase I enzymes.

Important Phase II enzymes include the glucuronic acid, glutathione, and sulfate systems. Glutathione is widely known to be a major antioxidant. Low levels of glutathione in the body are almost always a sign of illness, especially of poor immune function. How to correct low levels of glutathione will be discussed shortly in relation to the compound NAC.

Another Phase II enzyme of special importance is *glucuronic acid*. It is important for binding the toxic metabolites of the body's steroid hormones (estradiol, progesterone, and testosterone). Similarly, sulfate is active as a component in the compounds that prevent our bodies from reabsorbing the toxic substances that have already been processed for elimination from the body.

JESSE'S TIPS: TEN TOP ANTICANCER COMPOUNDS

Catechins—Found in most concentrated form in green tea, these are antioxidants and free radical scavengers. Chinese herbalism considers green tea to have an affinity for the liver.

Ellagic Acid—This polyphenol antioxidant and anticancer compound is most commonly found in certain fruits, especially strawberries, raspberries, and blackberries, but also in grapes and apples.

Glutathione—The mineral selenium's anticancer benefits depend in large part on its effect upon the body's production of glutathione, the powerful antioxidant detoxifier. Prostate cells that become cancerous typically have a defect in glutathione production. Good sources of glutathione and its building blocks are whey protein, asparagus, broccoli, and watermelon.

Indoles—Indole-3 carbinole, sulforophane, and calcium D-glucarate either stimulate the production of Phase II detoxification enzymes and/or prevent the reabsorption of toxic compounds the body has processed for elimination. Good sources are cruciferous vegetables such as broccoli, sprouts, and other cabbage family members.

Isoflavones—The best known of the isoflavones are genistein and daidzein from soybeans. Other good sources include red clover and various legumes. Isoflavones reduce the impact of toxic estrogen-like chemicals and may slow the division of cancer cells.

Lignans—These have anti-estrogen activity and can protect against hormonal cancers. The most concentrated source is flaxseeds.

Lycopene and other carotenoids—Lycopene is found in our daily diet, and has the best record in preventing the development of prostate cancer. Some other important carotenoids are cryptoxanthin, zeaxanthin, and lutein. Those supplementing the most common carotenoid, beta-carotene, should take extra vitamin E and should not consume alcohol. Lyco-Mato, a supplement I recommend, is particularly effective in treating prostate cancer. Developed in Israel, it contains a high level of lycopene.

Proanthocyanidins—These polyphenolic compounds are the primary active ingredients in grape seed extracts and are the most powerful protective compounds found in the red wine of the "French Paradox." These antioxidants help to protect the arteries, prevent the oxidation of LDL cholesterol, reduce blood pressure, and slow the invasion of cells by viruses. *In vitro* tests have shown protection against some forms of cancer and against cancer inducers.

Sulfur Compounds—Sulfur-containing compounds found in cruciferous vegetables and the allyl sulfides and related compounds found in garlic promote the action of glutathione in detoxification and antioxidant protection. These compounds improve immune function.

Terpenes—These antioxidants include limonoids, such as D-limonene, and technically include the carotenoids as well. D-limonene also activates the liver's Phase II enzyme system and is useful against some cancers.

Many of the benefits of the Phase II enzymes were discovered by studying the health benefits of eating certain vegetables. Remember broccoli? The anticancer benefits of broccoli and other cruciferous vegetables have been documented for many years. One study performed in Buffalo, New York, in the mid-1970s showed that the regular consumption of these vegetables dramatically reduced the incidence of colon and rectal cancer. Protection against these malignancies was dose-dependent—the more of these vegetables eaten, the more protection. Consuming several servings of cruciferous vegetables per week would go a very long way toward making these two forms of cancer endangered species in Americans.

Broccoli is a common item in the diets of those with very low rates of gastrointestinal tract cancers, ranging from those of the esophagus and stomach to those of the colon and rectum. Other studies have shown broccoli's protective effects against lung and breast cancers.

Much of the work done on broccoli and its cousins has focused upon the impact of compounds called "indoles" and "dithiolthiones." These compounds appear to activate the cellular Phase II enzymes described above. Even highly potent toxins, such as aflatoxin, cannot damage cellular DNA when these enzyme activators are fed to test animals. Indoles and dithiolthiones increase the amounts of glutathione and the enzymes that attach the glutathione to carcinogens. Broccoli's anticancer constituent, sulforaphane, which like the indoles and dithiolthiones, has been shown to raise the levels of Phase II enzymes.

If you wish to increase the effectiveness of Phase II enzymes, you must supply "building blocks" for these enzymes so that the body can make more of them, particularly glutathione. Probably the easiest way to do this with supplements is to take approximately 750 milligrams of N-acetyl-cysteine (NAC) per day, since glutathione itself is very poorly absorbed by most individuals. (Do not exceed this amount unless directed to do so by your physician.)

Other compounds seem to directly stimulate the production of Phase II compounds. Among these is indole-3-carbinol. The citrus oil extract D-limonene is already on the market and is a potent stimulant to Phase II enzyme production.

You may also look for concentrated whey protein, yet another source of building blocks for Phase II enzymes. Whey contains a particular set of fractions from milk that dramatically increase your body's ability to produce glutathione without the drawbacks true of other milk components when it comes to prostate cancer. Be sure your source of whey is ultrafiltered to remove toxins and hormone residues.

A second approach is to supplement with compounds that indirectly increase the building blocks of Phase II enzymes while performing other important functions in the body. Methyl donors such

---

JESSE'S TIPS: CANCER-FIGHTING SUPPLEMENTS

My usual suggestions to start with:
1. Antigen infused dialyzable bovine colostrum whey extract (further reference to this product will be AIDBCWE)
2. Coenzyme Q10, 100 milligrams three times daily
3. Shark liver oil, 2 soft gels twice daily
4. Vitamin D, 400 IU daily (not more than 800 IU total per day, unless directed)
5. Natural killer cell support complex, 1 tablespoon in vegetable juice or water, three times daily
6. Food state natural multivitamin/mineral tablets daily (regular maintenance formula)
7. Vitamin C, 1,000 milligrams three times daily

Supplements to support detoxification and immunomodulation:
1. Selenium, 200 to 400 micrograms daily
2. Gluthathione precursor complex, 2 capsules, three times daily
3. Calcium D-Glucarate, 200 to 400 milligrams daily
4. TMG (trimethylglycine), 500 to 750 milligrams daily
5. Isoflavones from soybeans, red clover, or other sources, as directed
6. D-limonene, 250 to 500 milligrams taken once or twice a day with meals
7. Green tea extract (40–60 percent catechins), 150 milligrams twice daily
8. Pine bark extract or grape seed extract (85–95 percent polyphenols), 150 milligrams twice daily
9. Flower pollen extract (water- and oil-soluble fractions), 2 tablets three times daily
10. Plant sterols and sterolins, 2 capsules three times daily
11. Barley grass concentrate (in pill or powder form), as directed, two or three times daily
12. Alpha-lipoic acid, 100 milligrams two or three times daily

as SAMe (S-adenosyl-methionine) and TMG (trimethylglycine) help to produce much of the body's cysteine for glutathione synthesis and also influence the availability of sulfate and the amino acid taurine. Methyl donors further protect the DNA through mechanisms that do not involve Phase II enzymes.

Finally, the supplement calcium D-glucarate improves the effectiveness of Phase II enzymes by preventing conjugated toxins from being freed by bacterial action in the intestines. Calcium D-glucarate blocks the unwanted actions of the enzymes that allow toxins to be reabsorbed into the body. Thus calcium D-glucarate might be viewed as the perfect partner for supplements that increase Phase II enzyme activity: it helps insure that the toxins that the Phase II enzymes have conjugated and bound for excretion do not somehow find their way back into our systems.

What Can Cause Prostate Cancer?

About 10 percent of all cases of prostate cancer are probably "inherited." Similarly, animal studies and other evidence suggest that artificial estrogens (xenoestrogens) in the environment in the form of pesticides, plastics, and other compounds, at least under laboratory conditions, readily cause prostate cancer. It is also clear that diet, lifestyle habits, and the environment contribute in some measure to the development of this cancer. We'll explore the risk factors for prostate cancer on the pages to follow.

A bit of caution is in order when interpreting some of these factors, especially those that may arise from dietary influences. Our ability to say with authority that prostate cancer is caused by a single factor in the diet, such as fat, is much weaker than is usually claimed. Unfortunately, our knowledge relies almost entirely upon studies that match the rates of prostate cancer in various groups to the diets followed by those groups. There are many problems with this approach, as we are, in essence, guessing at which factors should be studied and whether they are themselves causative or merely markers for something else either present or absent in the diet.

Here's a brief example to illustrate this point. In 1843, Stanislaw Tanchou (the French physician who discovered that autoimmune diseases are a distinct group of disorders) offered the first formula for predicting cancer risk. It was based on grain consumption and was found to accurately calculate cancer rates in major European cities. He calculated that the more grain consumed, the greater the rate of cancer. His paper, delivered to the Paris Medical Society, also mentioned that cancer and other "diseases of civilization" were almost never found in wild animal populations or among hunter-gatherers. This began a 100-year search for cancer in hunter-gatherers.

Today most epidemiologists would probably conclude that the higher rates of grain consumption in city dwellers found by Tanchou likely were true of relatively poor groups for whom grain constituted almost the entire diet. Monodiets are notorious for being linked to cancer. Therefore, we would say that Tanchou proved less that grain caused cancer than he proved that not eating other foods as well as grain (i.e., fruits, vegetables, adequate protein) might lead to elevated rates of cancer.

What, then, are the factors that likely lead to the development of prostate cancer?

Toxins in the Food Chain

Otto Warburg, the two-time Nobel Prize winner, believed that cancer cells were the response to either local or systemic reductions in available energy at the cellular level and that various toxins might be at work. Warburg's contemporary, Max Gerson, made a similar argument to the effect that a buildup of toxicity in the body, especially the liver, will lead to various functional and chemical alterations in the body. In both Gerson's model and Warburg's, cancerous cells, although not considered "healthy" or efficient under normal circumstances, represent a kind of "adaptation" to a degraded internal environment. The growth and spread of cancerous cells further degrades the internal environment, and the succeeding generations of cancer cells then adapt to changing conditions and become more virulent as they do so.

Our bodies produce a variety of toxic wastes routinely, and for this reason we possess well-developed enzymatic detoxification pathways. Unfortunately, these pathways can be overwhelmed when external sources of toxins are added to those found naturally in the food supply and to by-products of our own metabolism. Much of the material progress of the modern age has been accompanied by a rapid increase in the creation and release of toxic substances into the environment, often as growth promoters in agriculture.

Virtually all the derivatives from coal tar developed in the early years of this century were known even then to be carcinogens. Coal tar was an expensive source of raw materials from which to produce synthetic substances, however, and therefore not a great threat to the food chain. Oil, in contrast, is another matter entirely. It is plentiful and cheap. So are its accompanying hazards. Many or even most of the environmental toxins derived from petroleum are classifiable as (xeno)estrogens because they mimic certain effects of estrogen, the so-called female hormone.

HORMONE MIMICS AND ENDOCRINE DISRUPTORS

Xenoestrogens are environmental—and usually synthetic—compounds that mimic one or more of estrogen's actions in the body. These compounds are also called "endocrine distruptors" because they disturb the body's normal hormonal balance. Most of these compounds are made from oil, coal, and/or are chemicals synthesized with the elements chlorine and fluorine. Combining tiny amounts of two or more of these compounds together greatly magnifies their effects to disrupt normal growth, behavior, and reproduction; they are implicated in many cancers. Common estrogen mimics include:

- alkyphenols (used in many detergents, pesticides, and personal care products; transformed by bacteria into the estrogen mimic nonylphenol and related compounds)
- DDT and other pesticides
- dioxin
- chlorinated/fluorinated hydrocarbons
- methoxychlor (pesticide)
- PCBs (polychlorinated biphenyls)
- plasticizers (used in some plastic wraps and containers)

These synthetic estrogens appear to be significantly represented in both male and female hormonally induced cancers, i.e., prostate cancer and breast cancer. Few researchers have looked for a direct connection between synthetic or xenoestrogens and prostate cancer, but an estimated 90 percent of all women with breast cancer suffer from abnormally high levels of estrogens in their systems. Similarly, biopsies of breast tissue from women with breast cancer typically show between 300 and 600 percent greater contamination with PCBs (polychlorinated biphenyls) than do biopsies from women without cancer. Synthetic estrogen (xenoestrogen) sources consist of many or even most pesticides and herbicides, plastics (including food wraps), industrial chemicals now common in ground water supplies, etc.

Does this mean that the plastic wrapper for your ground meat purchased at the local supermarket may be releasing its xenoestrogenic payload into your burgers and meat loaf? You'd better believe it! Lots of other common wrappings and containers do the same. This is especially a problem when fats and fat-soluble foods, like cheese, are wrapped in plastics.

Men must rely on less direct evidence than is currently available with regard to breast cancer. As mentioned earlier, the rate of testicular cancer, a cancer normally found in men under thirty-five years of age, has increased sharply in recent decades. Indeed, over the last fifty years testicular cancer—an easily recognized cancer—has increased 100 percent in white males and 200 percent in black males.

Animal experiments have shown clearly that the simultaneous treatment of male animals with both testosterone and estrogen (in the form of estradiol-17-beta) quickly leads to the development of precancerous prostate lesions in *all* of the experimental animals, whereas treatment with testosterone alone did not have this effect. *Hence it is hard to avoid the conclusion that environmental estrogens may play a very large role in the development of prostate cancer.*

What can you do to lessen the burden of xenoestrogens in your diet? Quite a bit, actually. In my own household, we buy organically grown fruits and vegetables, both because they tend to taste better and because they are free of pesticides, herbicides, etc. Also, you might be surprised how many foods can be purchased in bulk and stored without being wrapped in plastic wraps and the like. As for milk products and meats, here one must be especially careful, as growth hormones are used routinely in the raising of animals and in the dairy industry. I try not to put my family at risk, and I advise the same caution to others.

A number of authorities have urged men with prostate cancer or family histories of prostate cancer to add large amounts of soy products and fiber to the diet. Soy products contain what are known as *phytoestrogens*. These very weak estrogens of plant origin can be eaten to block the effects of synthetic estrogens and even to reduce the effects of the estrogens produced in our own bodies; this is the chief virtue of the soybean in prostate cancer. Fiber binds to hormones in the intestinal tract and prevents their reabsorption. It also prevents the unwanted action by bacteria on these compounds and then the reabsorption of toxic by-products.

Testosterone, DHT, and Vasectomies

As mentioned earlier, African-American men have rates of prostate cancer roughly 40 percent higher than those found in Caucasian-American men, or a 1 in 9 chance of developing prostate cancer versus a 1 in 11 chance for white males. One suspected reason is that black men do have higher levels of circulating testosterone than those of white men of the same age. In fact, these levels are roughly 15 percent higher than those of young white men. This explanation assumes, of course, that testosterone levels largely control the incidence of prostate cancer, which is yet to be proven.

European and American men, on the other hand, have higher rates of prostate cancer than do Japanese men, much in line with the comparison between black and white male testosterone levels. It has been found that Dutch men, for instance, have higher testosterone levels than do their Japanese counterparts and that American men have higher levels of the testosterone metabolite called DHT than do Japanese men.

This line of evidence is suggestive, but of what? Both diet and emotional factors (stress) influence testosterone levels. Blacks who are vegetarians have lower testosterone levels than those who are not. It has been shown experimentally that men who are put in positions where they are more "successful," more athletically active, or more emotionally or physically *aggressive* also have higher testosterone levels. How much of the difference in testosterone levels between young blacks and young whites in America is a reflection of culture and sociological factors and how much is a reflection of genetics? Moreover, prostate cancer typically develops and becomes significant only as testosterone levels are *falling,* and especially as the ratio of testosterone to estrogen has dramatically declined. This would seem to indicate that levels of total testosterone may have little relevance to the development of prostate cancer.

This last point is taken up at some length in a later chapter and in an appendix that discusses other issues of the prostate. However, the evidence does not seem to support the conclusion that testosterone causes prostate cancer, but rather that testosterone *in the presence of estrogen,* and perhaps *especially in the presence of xenoestrogens,* may increase the risk of prostate cancer. Animal experiments have shown that simply giving testosterone to male animals does not necessarily increase the rate of prostate cancer, but that giving *both* testosterone *and* estrogen will cause prostate cancer in 100 percent of the animals tested. The increased level of estrogen relative to testosterone affects how these hormones bind to prostate cells, which has unfortunate consequences.

Vasectomies are another point of controversy. In two large studies, men with vasectomies had, respectively, a 66 percent and a 56 percent greater risk of prostate cancer than did men without vasectomies. Nevertheless, a later panel of experts brought together by the National Institutes of Health concluded that there is no elevated risk of prostate cancer in those with vasectomies. It may be that men who undergo this operation have higher rates of detection, rather than higher rates of incidence. Yet, it is also known that there are slightly higher rates of lung cancer in men who have undergone vasectomies, and the argument for better detection would not hold here. The jury is still out.

Red Meat, Fat, and Sugar

The issues of whether red meat, fat, and sugar lead to a greater incidence of prostate cancer and to a greater death rate among those who already have cancer are controversial. Recommendations in this area are also often contradictory. For example, those who suggest that fat intake should be kept below 15 percent of total calories will also typically suggest that fatty fish should be reduced or eliminated from the diet. Yet Japanese studies have shown that prostate cancer levels are lower in men who eat more fish.

Let's start with the issues of red meat and fat. Most studies have found positive correlations between the consumption of red meat and prostate cancer. Many studies, as well, have found strong correlations between high-fat diets, especially animal fat diets, and prostate cancer. However, at least in the case of fat in the diet, other studies have found either no relationship or, at most, a very weak one. One very large and thorough study came to the following conclusions:

> Total prostate cancer was unrelated to total fat, saturated fat, monosatu-rated fat, and linoleic acid. The consumption of animal fat, especially fat from red meat, was associated with an increased risk of advanced cancers (stage C and D and fatal cancers). (Giovannucci, E. et al., *Journal of the National Cancer Institute*, 1993)

Two important factors are at work here. First, the estrogen-like toxins just described tend to collect in animal products, especially red meat. Today it is quite difficult to distinguish data regarding meat consumption from the estrogenic toxins that can collect in meat products. And remember, the plastic wrap used to present meat in the display case at your local market is yet another source of estrogenic contaminants.

Worse yet, American agribusiness commonly uses a variety of synthetic estrogens to cause weight gain in animals. This practice is so pervasive that the European Union has now refused to accept even supposedly "hormone free" or "organically grown" American beef because tests showed that more than a third of the exported "hormone free" beef contained hormone residues! The best recommendation for meat eaters is to buy and consume only certified organically grown meats. Another idea is to focus on meats from animals that are not usually given growth hormones, such as lamb and buffalo.

A second factor hidden in the statistics on fat consumption and prostate cancer is that this data may be a better indicator of what is *not* eaten, rather than of what is. Remember the case of the Frenchman who believed that eating excessive amounts of grain caused cancer? In modern diets, especially in the United States, those who eat the most fat typically eat the fewest vegetables. Was it the consumption of the red meat and its fat, or omitting vegetables, that was most significant? Diets that lack adequate levels of vegetables can cause severe problems because they lack antioxidants, free radical scavengers, and Phase I and II enzymes for detoxification.

Sugar is another proposed risk factor for prostate cancer. This is in part because an increased level of sugar consumption increases the risk of obesity, and obesity is a risk factor for prostate cancer. It is also true that insulin, the hormone that controls blood sugar levels, is connected to strong risk factors for prostate and other cancers.

In addition, sugar in its various forms (sucrose and fructose) dampens immune response. Lactose, fructose, and perhaps other sugars have also been linked to elevations in ischemic heart disease, a major health risk in men. Finally, concentrated sources of sugars, like concentrated sources of animal fats, are usually found in diets

---

JESSE'S TIPS: BEWARE SUGAR SOURCES

Sugar comes in many forms and is often "hidden" in foods. For instance, "fruit" yogurts usually have very substantial amounts of sugar in the "fruit" portion. Soft drinks are another tremendous source of sugar in the diet. Many peanut and other nut butters, even some canned meats, now contain added sugars. Also, the more refined and processed any carbohydrate is—instant oatmeal, for instance, instead of old-fashioned rolled oats—the more it acts in the body like sugar. Beware! Sugars and sugar sources include:

beet sugar	honey
cane sugar	lactose
corn syrup	maltose
dextrine	maple syrup
dextrose	maltodextrine
dried fruits	molasses and dehydrated molasses
fructose	saccharose
grape sugar	sucrose

It is very important to read the ingredients lists on prepared foods. Sugars are usually there in the "fine print."

skimpy in the consumption of vegetables and fresh whole fruits (as opposed to juices, which are mostly sugar).

A primary need of the patient with prostate cancer is to improve the efficiency of his body's detoxification pathways. As a protein source, fish is as beneficial as red meat. Fats and sugars should be sharply reduced in favor of foods that support detoxification.

Milk and IGF-1, the Issue of Calcium

In January 1998, the journal *Science* reported that a study of 15,000 men found that those whose blood levels of insulin-like growth factor-1 (IGF-1) were high were four times more likely to develop prostate cancer than those whose blood levels were low. IGF-1 is a peptide (a small protein molecule) involved in regulating the effects of growth hormone. It is a powerful stimulant to growth in cancerous tissues, as well as in normal tissues. Significantly, IGF-1 levels are usually elevated *seven years* in advance of PSA scores. High IGF-1 levels are markers for any cancer, not just prostate cancer. Nevertheless, the mere fact that IGF-1 has such predictive capacity so many years in advance of any organic manifestation is significant and also a piece of evidence for the view put forth by researchers such as Warburg and Gerson.

Milk consumption has been strongly linked to the development of prostate cancer. The risk factors are highest with regard to the calcium and the nonfat portions of the milk (skim milk and nonfat milk). Several theories have been put forth to explain this data. One is that milk contains one or more substances that act similarly to IGF-1 in our bodies. Milk, after all, is designed to speed and support the growth of a young animal. IGF-1-like fractions are proteins, so drinking skim and/or nonfat milk does no good in avoiding these.

There is another antimilk theory that need not entirely exclude the first. It suggests that the calcium in milk inhibits the conversion of vitamin D from the form in which it is found in the blood to the form in which it can suppress prostate cancer. For instance, in a 1999 Harvard study involving 47,000 men, those who consumed 2,000 milligrams of calcium per day were twice as likely to develop prostate cancer as those who consumed only 1,000 milligrams per day.

JESSE'S TIPS: FOODS TO RESTRICT AND AVOID

Restrict or eliminate animal products—
red meats, animal fats, dairy products.

Restrict or eliminate processed and artificial products—
refined flours, prepared cereals, canned goods, prepared or "instant" foods, preserved foods, foods containing dyes/colorings and preservatives, foods containing artificial sweeteners and flavorings.

Restrict fats, both saturated fats and oils from seed grains—
avoid omega-6 fatty acids (found in corn, cotton, safflower and soybean oils), and eliminate trans-fatty acids (found in margarine and hydrogenated fats).

Restrict seed grain products—
cut back or eliminate wheat and corn products.

Eliminate all sugars—
sugars are often hidden; consult the tips on sugars.

Eliminate unhealthful beverages—
caffeine, alcohol, soft drinks of all kinds (including "diet" drinks).

Deficiencies and Imbalances: Vitamins D and A

As you have seen, both too much and too little of otherwise essential nutrients can increase one's risk of contracting prostate cancer. Even beneficial nutrients can interact in unforeseen ways.

The protective effects of vitamin D are supported by considerable data. As pointed out with regard to the elevated rates of prostate cancer in black American males, a reduced ability to produce vitamin D from sunlight may be significant. This is found to be true in white males as well as in black males. Prostate cancer rates rise as one moves from the sunny Southwest to the cloudy Northeast, and it is a simple matter to find a protective influence based upon the number of sunny days enjoyed each year! Of course, it still could also be that the mood-brightening effects of the sun are at work, as well. . . .

JESSE'S TIPS: FOODS TO ADD TO YOUR DIET

Always try to eat only organically grown foods.

Special Protectors—
Organic ground flaxseeds, soybean protein concentrate, walnuts, essential fatty acids, broccoli, cabbage and other cabbage-family vegetables.

Meat alternatives—
Fish, organically raised free–range chicken and turkey, tempeh and other soy products.

Brightly colored vegetables and fruits—
five or more servings of dark green and highly colored vegetables every day; two whole fruits (not juice) per day.

Healthful alternatives to wheat—
aduki beans, amaranth, brown rice, barley, beets, lentils, millet, mung beans, quinoa, soy products (especially fermented soy foods), sweet potatoes and yams.

Oils—
For salads, use walnut, extra virgin olive, hazelnut and other nut oils; for cooking, use extra virgin olive oil.

Flavorings—
curry, garlic, ginger, onion, turmeric, aged garlic extract, fresh and dried herbs.

Beverages—
green tea, herbal teas, plenty of pure water, fresh vegetable juices.

Vitamin A deficiency is another factor often linked to elevated rates of prostate cancer. Vitamin A is especially important for the health of epithelial tissues, from which prostate cancer develops. In large epidemiological trials, this vitamin comes out as a strong risk-reducing factor.

Related to vitamin A are the brightly colored red, orange, and yellow pigments, or *carotenoids,* found in fruits and vegetables. Many of these carotenoids can be transformed into vitamin A by the body.

The most protective carotenoid for prostate health appears to be *lycopene*, the red coloring matter found in tomatoes. Tomato dishes comprise a large portion of the diets of Italians and Greeks, and studies typically find that prostate cancer risk in southern Europeans is half that of central Europeans. To be effectively absorbed, lycopene from fresh raw tomatoes must be cooked. Cooking tomatoes in sauces that contain olive oil or another fat dramatically improves the availability of lycopene for assimilation during digestion.

Among their many other good effects, lycopene inhibits prostate cancer cell proliferation induced by IGF-1. As another, unrelated benefit, lycopenes protect the LDL cholesterol from the harmful oxidative process that leads to atherosclerosis, blood vessel plaque formation, heart attacks, and strokes. So for the Number 1 and Number 2 killers in North America, lycopene is a friend indeed, so . . . *mangia!*

These are the nutrients found commonly in diets that have most closely been identified with good prostate health. However, good health and success against prostate cancer require sound nutrition in general, not just prostate nutrition. A healthy prostate cannot exist in an unhealthy body.

JESSE'S TIPS: BEST LYCOPENE FOOD SOURCES

Amounts in milligrams of lycopene per 100 grams of foodstuff; total lycopene content can be misleading inasmuch as cooking with oil dramatically improves assimilation. For example, tomato juice is a poor lycopene source compared with tomato paste and sauce despite its higher relative content of this carotenoid.

Food	Amount	Food	Amount
Ketchup	9.9	Watermelon	4.1
Tomato juice	8.6	Papaya	3.7
Tomato paste	6.5	Tomatoes, cooked	3.7
Tomato sauce	6.2	Grapefruit, pink	3.4
Guava	5.4	Guava juice	3.3
		Apricots, dried	0.9

CHAPTER TWO

Detecting Prostate Cancer

I am more than ever convinced that biochemistry and metabolic science will be victorious in healing degenerative diseases, including cancer, if the *whole body* or the *whole metabolism* will be addressed and not just the symptoms.
—Max Gerson, M.D. in *Has Dr. Max Gerson a True Cancer Cure?*

Case Study: Ken V. is a 37-year-old Wall Street commodity trader with newly diagnosed (one-year) metastatic prostate cancer. It was found only as a result of his persistent complaints of back pain. He was started on triple androgen blockade, but didn't tolerate the side effects and sought another approach. I placed him on PC SPES, shark liver oil, flaxseed oil, ADBCWE, Iscucin, selenium, vitamin C, lycopene, vitamin D, glutathione precursor complex, Co-Q10, shark liver oil, and a food state natural multivitamin/mineral. He made a number of significant lifestyle changes, including giving up cigarettes, alcohol, coffee, fast food, and late-night parties. He started to meditate and took a wood sculpture course to help balance the stress of his livelihood. Over a period of five months, his PSA dropped from 345 to 1.2. He is still in counseling and views his cancer as a "gift" that opened him up to all the richness in life that he was missing.

Commentary: Prostate cancer is a great impersonator. Although in this man's case it gave rise to seemingly unrelated symptoms, cancer of the prostate can remain remarkably inconspicuous for many years. Aside from the fact that this cancer typically grows slowly, its effects upon the structure and the functions of the prostate are usually not dramatic until its late stages. Only a small part of the total area of the prostate lies adjacent to the urethra, and unless the cancerous part of the prostate just happens to be in this portion, even a quite enlarged prostate may not affect urination.

The Prostate-Specific Antigen (PSA) and Other Tests

Physicians use four primary tests to diagnose prostate cancer and a wide range of others to gauge the extent of the cancer. Three are noninvasive, including the digital rectal exam (DRE), the PSA test, and the transrectal ultrasound test. The biopsy of the prostate is the last, and most invasive, test.

Digital Rectal Examination (DRE)— The One-Finger Salute

The digital rectal examination is exactly what its name suggests: the manual palpation of the prostate gland. To perform the test, a physician puts on a glove and inserts the index finger into the patient's rectum. Only a very thin wall separates the prostate from the lower end of the large intestine, and it is possible to probe the prostate by feeling it through this wall. By moving the gloved finger along the intestinal wall, the doctor can feel both lobes of the gland. This examination establishes several facts, including the prostate's size, shape, hardness, and degree of irregularity.

A healthy prostate is roughly the size of a walnut, with a regular shape and smooth surface. It is firm, but not hard. Enlargement can result from a number of conditions, and is usually noncancerous. Too soft a texture may indicate inflammation. Too hard a texture, irregularities, and/or the presence of hard nodules may indicate cancer.

Of the primary screening tests for prostate cancer, the DRE is the *least* reliable. Leaving aside the awkward fact that healthy prostates may naturally feel quite different when probed due to the uniqueness of the individual's prostate, the test has some recognized limitations. For one thing, a tumor must already be about a cubic centimeter in size before it can be felt. Given the fact that the entire prostate gland is only the size of a walnut, a tumor half the size of a peanut is already quite significant. This slow-growing cancer may be present for many years before it reaches a size at which it can be felt as a bump or node. Another weakness of the DRE is that cancerous tumors may begin on the side of the prostate that is not accessible from the rectum. In fact, most cancers begin on the posterior (back) of the prostate. Finally, a man can suffer from more than one prostate condition. One can suffer from an enlarged benign prostate and still have prostate cancer at the same time. The additional tissue under these conditions will make detecting tumor nodules even more difficult.

Current estimates are that less than half of all cases of prostate cancer are detectable by rectal examination. On the other hand, when bumps or nodules are found, at least half of these are not cancerous. These conditions are called "false negatives" and "false positives," that is, cases in which a clean bill of health is given to someone who does have cancer, and cases in which someone who does not have cancer is diagnosed as having it. The PSA test was introduced, in part, in the hopes of reducing both figures.

Prostate-Specific Antigen (PSA) Test

The prostate-specific antigen is an enzyme produced only by prostate cells and is measurable in trace amounts in the bloodstream. This enzyme is produced by the prostate as long as testosterone is present. The general idea behind the PSA test is that the PSA count rises as the quantity of prostate tissue increases. Cancerous prostate tissues tend to release at least ten times more of the antigen on a gram-per-gram basis than do normal prostate tissues due, in part, to the fact that cancerous tissues block drainage of PSA into the urethra. Test scores in a healthy individual normally will vary somewhat because of test limitations, but as a rule, safe scores are below 4.0 ng/ml, i.e., below 4 nanograms (billionths of a gram) per milliliter of blood. Scores between 4.0 and 10.0 ng/ml indicate a potential problem, and scores above 10.0 strongly suggest that cancer is present. Test results can usually be had within two to four days.

The PSA test is at least twice as accurate as the DRE, yet it, too, has several drawbacks. For instance, some men have larger prostates than do others, and the same is also true across racial groups, e.g., Japanese men typically have smaller prostates and lower PSA scores than do Dutch men. Safe PSA scores must also be matched to a man's age. Some authorities estimate that men aged 50 years old should consider PSA scores of 2.5 and below safe (some would say below 3.0), whereas men aged 70–75 should consider scores below 4.5 to be safe (some would say below 6.0 or even 6.5), that is, not even in a "gray" area. Moreover, many factors besides cancer will increase PSA scores. Scores may be increased by BPH, prostate infections, sexual activity within 10 days, medical examinations of the prostate, and so forth. And if you've had a biopsy, your PSA score may increase fifty-fold for two weeks or more! So be sure to delay that PSA for a few weeks after your biopsy for a more accurate score.

False negative PSA scores in men whose scores are seemingly normal are found in up to 40 percent of men with prostate cancer. That's a very high number! Similarly, almost two-thirds of positive results turn out to be false alarms if the scores are between 2.5 and 10 ng/ml. The difficulty here is the range: Men with scores of 1.8 ng/ml or below can have prostate cancer, and 40 percent of men with PSA scores below 4 ng/mg may have prostate cancer that is localized in the prostate gland. PSA scores over a period of time are much better indicators of prostate health than are individual tests, as are sudden increases in PSA scores. With PSA scores above 10 ng/ml, there is much less ambiguity.

Refinements of the PSA test have been proposed to improve the accuracy of the test. Most promising in this regard is the development of the "free PSA" test. When a fraction of the circulating PSA is found attached to other proteins in the serum (the clear portion of the blood), it is said to be "bound." The rest is unbound, or "free." Tests have determined that men with prostate cancer have lower percentages of free PSA in proportion to total PSA than do men with noncancerous prostates. Hence, the lower the level of free PSA to total PSA, the less likely it is that the PSA score reflects a noncancerous development, such as BPH. It is more likely that a high PSA reading is indicative of cancer. This refinement of the PSA test is most important for those with readings of 4.0 to 10.0 ng/ml. It can help reduce the number of false negative results and help determine if a biopsy should be performed. If your regular PSA is higher than 4.0, I urge you to take the "free PSA" test as a backup.

There is general agreement in recent trials that about one-third of all men who have PSA scores of greater than 4.0 ng/ml have prostate cancer. There is also broad agreement that the free-to-total PSA test will reduce unnecessary invasive procedures based on false positive results by about 30 percent. Even more refinements have been proposed to further improve the power of the PSA test. These should become available in the near future.

Transrectal Ultrasound (TRUS)

Only if the DRE or the PSA test turns up a problem will the physician plan other, more invasive procedures. Transrectal ultrasound (TRUS) examination is conducted by placing a small probe into the rectum to emit high-frequency sound waves. These sound waves pass through the wall of the rectum (hence, "transrectal"), strike the prostrate, and return as "echoes" to the probe to give an "image" of the gland. A computer transforms the signals into visual images for display on a monitor.

The TRUS takes only about twenty minutes, and can provide a picture of cancerous nodules, but is increasingly being used to guide the doctor in performing a biopsy. The TRUS alone has a number of limitations; for example, it may be unable to distinguish between cancerous and noncancerous nodules.

Biopsy

The final step in the diagnosis of prostate cancer is the biopsy of tissue from the prostate for examination under a microscope. In many more modern procedures, the TRUS itself is used to facilitate the biopsy. Biopsy needles are designed with hollow cores and are spring-loaded into special "guns" that can be directed at small areas of the prostate through the wall of the rectum. Each needle retrieves a core of tissue when it is withdrawn.

Only by retrieving actual tissue samples can the doctor be completely certain whether an abnormality is cancerous. Usually, a pattern of samples are taken from the prostate to represent each section of the gland. Microscopic examination of the tissue then allows for an analysis of the nature and the virulence of the cancer. Cancer cells are given a Gleason score, a measure of the degree of abnormality observed in the cancer.

Other Tests

If cancer is present, several other tests may be run. A *bone scan* may be performed to determine if the cancer has metastasized to the bones, especially those near the prostate. The bone scan is a special form of X-ray in which a mildly radioactive dye is first injected into the system. This dye collects in the bones and makes them appear more clearly on film. Cancerous tissues concentrate the dye and thus show up as "hot spots" when viewed. Unfortunately, other forms of damage, such as breaks and arthritis, will also appear. To clarify results, bone scan readings are often compared with those from other tests, such as those from the MRI.

An especially popular diagnostic tool is the *magnetic resonance imaging* (MRI) test. Instead of X-rays, this device employs powerful magnetic fields that elicit distinguishable signals from different tissues and cells. A computer transforms the data into cross-sectional images of tissues and organs. These images are particularly valuable in showing the spinal cord and the brain, and allow more specific interpretations of the state of the bones than do simple bone scan results.

Akin to the MRI is the *computerized axial tomography* (CAT) scan, also called the *computerized tomography,* or CT scan. The CAT scan provides yet another computer-generated cross-sectional view of tissues and organs, but this one is built from multiple X-rays taken in a 360-degree rotation of the body. A dye may be ingested or injected to enhance the image. The CAT scan is performed primarily to pinpoint cancer sites before radiation therapy.

One other test frequently done after a positive biopsy is the *pro-*

static acid phosphatase (PAP) test. This compound is usually above normal levels in men whose prostate cancer is spreading, and can be checked in blood, urine, or prostate secretions. It is not an accurate test on its own, as the PAP can be elevated by BPH and a number of other conditions, some drugs, or a rectal exam.

There are other "new kids on the block." One of the most promising is the ProstaScint test for tracing prostate cancer tumors. It is yet another whole-body imaging scan, and it promises to be the most accurate of these scans for this purpose.

Grading: Gleason Scores and DNA Ploidy Analysis

If cancer cells are discovered by the biopsy, these cells are further examined to determine how aggressively the cancer can be expected to behave. By far the most popularly accepted yardstick currently for this purpose is one developed by a physician named Gleason. A Gleason score, or grade, is assigned on the basis of the cells' shape in relation to that of normal cells of the same type, the degree of abnormality of the gland itself, and the tumor's boundary in relationship to adjoining noncancerous tissue.

Grading is made on a scale of 1 to 5 by comparing the nature of the cancerous cells to normal cells. If the cancer cells closely resemble the norm for their tissue type (this is known as being "well-differentiated"), are evenly spaced in relation to each other, and form a compact mass with a defined margin between tumor and nontumor tissue areas, the pathologist gives a grade of 1. As the cells resemble normal cells less and less, becoming more jagged and less compact, and progressively invade the surrounding tissue, the score increases to a maximum of 5, at which point there is no resemblance to normal prostate cells.

As the pathologist views his sample of cells, he identifies the two most common cell patterns as the *primary* and the *secondary* patterns. The scores of these two patterns are added together to yield the Gleason score. The lowest (and safest) score is $1 + 1 = 2$ and the highest is $5 + 5 = 10$. Scores of 4 and below describe a "well-differentiated" cancer. Scores of 5 to 6 represent "moderate differentiation," and scores of 7 to 10 represent a "poorly differentiated" cancer. Traditionally, as the score rises, the prognosis worsens.

Several other techniques have been developed to try to predict more accurately how a given case of prostate cancer will fare. Aside from the Gleason score, a growing number of my colleagues and I are now using a technique called *DNA Ploidy Analysis*. The starting point, once again, is cells obtained by biopsy. These cells are then exposed to a fluorescent dye that stains the cellular DNA. Next, the degree to which these cells fluoresce upon exposure to a special light is measured, and this data is used to determine the number of complete sets of chromosomes in the cells. Since both the growth rate of the cancer and its likelihood of metastasis can be roughly calculated from DNA ploidy data, I believe this is a very useful test that may even be more revealing than the Gleason score.

There are still other tests designed to determine if the cancer has spread. The most common are *reverse transcriptase polymerase chain reaction* (RT-PCR), *serum acid phosphatase* (ACP), and *alkaline phosphatase* (ALP). The scores from these various tests are guides or yardsticks to make decisions regarding forms of treatment.

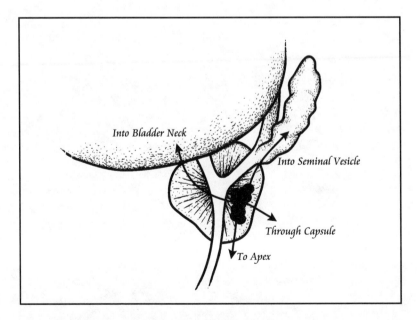

Figure 2. The Early Spread of Prostate Cancer. Prostate cancer quickly invades the surrounding tissues once the prostate capsule has been breached.

However, a high score is not the end of the world any more than a low score is a signal for complacency.

Finally, doctors not only *grade* prostate cancer, but also give it *stages*, usually based upon the international *TNM standard*. TNM stands for tumor, nodes, and metastasis, and there are substages as well as stages. The TNM system is merely a shorthand description of the extent of the original tumor, the status of the nodes of the local lymphatic system, and whether there is metastasis to other more distant parts of the body. Because the TNM staging system is quite elaborate, a patient's score is best discussed in person with his doctor.

CHAPTER THREE

Destroying the Cancer

A later chapter will describe in detail not only most of the treatments available for prostate cancer, but how these treatments are best orchestrated to provide maximum benefits. However, precisely because an integrated approach is not the norm, it is useful to begin with some of the pros and cons of the more usual forms of treatment.

Conventional Treatments

Watchful Waiting

One approach to a diagnosis of prostate cancer is to practice what is termed "watchful waiting." For many men diagnosed with prostate cancer, watchful waiting may prove to be more appropriate than any form of radical intervention. Some 80 percent of all diagnoses of prostate cancer are in men aged 65 years old and above, and prostate cancer often grows very slowly. In the judgment of some physicians, surgery and other radical treatments are not warranted if the patient's life expectancy is less than 10 years. In such cases, surgery probably will neither prolong life nor improve the quality of life.

To be sure, watchful waiting does not mean that one does nothing. A diagnosis of prostate cancer can be a wake-up call to change eating habits, increase levels of physical activity, and examine the nature of one's emotional responses to life.

Radical Prostatectomy

If the cancer is discovered before it has moved out of the prostate proper, it is possible to "cure" the cancer by removing the prostate. Unfortunately, even with this radical procedure performed at a relatively early stage in the development of the cancer, at least 20 percent of surgeries turn out to be failures due to cancer cells that may have escaped the surgeon's knife. Some experts put the failure rate much higher. Radical prostatectomy makes sense as a therapeutic intervention only in generally healthy and relatively young men, usually at ages of 55 and below, because the risks and drawbacks of the procedure are not warranted if life expectancy is less than 10 years.

The surgery can require a hospital stay of up to a week, bed rest at home of up to 10 weeks, and full recovery may take 6 months. Complications include incontinence, impotence, blood loss, and complications arising from the surgery itself, such as injuries to the rectum and the urethra. This is considered major surgery, with all the possible complications inherent in such an operation. Radical prostatectomy may be an option for the younger man, but it is certainly not one without risks or with guarantees.

Radical prostatectomy's popularity is, however, slowly increasing throughout the nation. Detection of prostate cancer is now possible at an earlier age. In addition, one of the primary drawbacks of the surgery, complete impotence, can be avoided by using newer techniques that can spare the nerves running along either side of the prostate. By some estimates, as many as 90 percent of men under age 50 when they undergo radical prostatectomy may regain their potency as the surgery is now performed.

Chemotherapy

Chemotherapy forms used with other cancers have not been successful with prostate cancer and are not recommended. All the usual side effects are present, but at this time, there is no increase in survival rates.

Radiation Therapies and Cryotherapy

There are two common forms of radiation therapy for prostate cancer. In one, a focused beam of X-rays is directed at the site(s) of the cancer, and the procedure is repeated for several weeks running. However, only very early stage cancers can be "cured" by this technique, and even then the cure rate is probably not more than 20 percent. Some studies have shown that two years after treatment, tumors can still be found in as high as 93 percent of patients! Even more unfortunate is the fact that in the 80 percent of patients not cured by this treatment, the procedure appears to cause the cancer to *increase* its rate of growth!

Aside from hopes for a cure, the only other reason to use radiation beam therapy is to improve some aspects of already metastasized cancers. In some cases in which the cancer has spread to the bones near the prostate, radiation beams can reduce pain and the rate of subsequent fractures. In both of these uses, the side effects are much the same, ranging from fatigue, impotence, nausea, and vomiting to painful urination to permanent (and quite painful) damage to the rectum and the bladder. However, Cancer Treatment Centers of America use a special reduced-dose external beam radiotherapy with conformal blocking that gives excellent results with much fewer side effects (see below).

A second form of radiation therapy, called *interstitial brachytherapy*, involves the implantation of numerous radioactive "seeds" into the prostate gland which are left in place and frequently cause numerous side effects to the bladder, urethra, and rectum. *Cryotherapy*, instead of radioactive pellets, places very low temperature needles temporarily into the cancerous portions of the gland to freeze the tumor(s). Neither of these techniques has been subject to enough long-term studies to determine a cure rate. However, I personally prefer to avoid any invasive therapy when I can achieve a high success rate without them.

It's not very often that I get excited about a hospital-based therapy. However, Cancer Treatment Centers of America (CTCA 1-800-

FOR-HELP) has begun a pioneering prostate cancer treatment program called High-Dose Rate Temporary Brachytherapy that *is* exciting! Essentially painless, it involves gently placing 2 millimeter diameter (tiny) plastic catheters into the prostate gland and then giving four radiation treatments through these catheters over a 30-hour period. The catheters are then removed and *nothing* is left in the prostate gland. The dose is computer driven by the shape of the prostate and the exact location of the cancer. Thus the side effects are reduced. The outcome is generally brighter due to the radiation oncologist's ability to focus and isolate the radiation dose. This "smart-bomb" approach obviously makes the most sense, in terms of radiation therapy.

If a patient has a small, localized, early prostate cancer, I may recommend this course of treatment. Then I would start to vigorously wake up the immune system to minimize the possibility of any recurrence. See the Resource Section for further information about this exciting, new, and innovative therapy.

Hormonal Therapy

Hormonal therapy is often the treatment of choice once the cancer has metastasized. The basic principle behind current hormonal therapy is that most cells in prostate cancer tumors are "sensitive" to the androgenic (male sex) hormone testosterone. Although not a cure for prostate cancer, hormonal therapy can usually reduce the size of tumors and inhibit their growth for up to two to three years. Some men may, however, find their tumors become "refractory," meaning that they begin to grow again. In part, tumors that are refractory to hormonal therapy become increasingly made up of androgen-insensitive cells that have replaced the original androgen-sensitive ones—sometimes within a year of initiating therapy.

Hormonal therapy is really a hormonal blockade. Medications such as Lupron, Casodex, or Zoladex can radically reduce the production of testosterone by the testicles. (The same could be achieved by the removal of the testes, or *orchiectomy*, but relatively few men go this route.) The adrenal glands, as well as the testicles, produce some androgenic hormones, and therefore a more complete treatment requires the use of a second drug, usually a Flutamide. The prescription of this combination of drugs is called *combined hormonal blockade* (CHB) or *total androgen blockade* (TAB). Sometimes these are also called combination hormonal therapy (CHT). Quite a few variants on this theme are currently being practiced, and the list of drugs is in rapid flux. Currently I like, and on occasion use, Proscar, Flutamide, and Zoladex together with PC SPES. Recently, CHB has been combined with radiation therapy with improved results. Also, new forms of antiandrogenic therapies are constantly being developed. Side effects for these treatments include sexual impotence, nausea, anemia, and hot flashes.

When I use CHB, I prefer to use it as *intermittent hormonal therapy* (IHT). IHT is combination hormonal therapy that is applied during intervals, instead of on a continuous basis. The idea behind IHT

STANDARD PROSTATE CANCER TREATMENTS

Antiandrogens bicalutamide (Casodex®) cyproterone flutamide (Eulexin®)	Prevents DHT from binding to its prostate cell receptors.
Estrogens Diethylstilbesterol (DES)	Inhibit LHRH release from the hypothalamus.
LHRH Analogs luprolide (Lupron Depot®) goserelin acetate (Zoladex®) nafarelin (Synarel®)	Stimulate excessive LHRH production leading ultimately to feedback-induced cessation of LHRH production; causes hypothalamus to stop its signal for the production of LH.
5AR Inhibitors finasteride (Proscar®)	Inhibit 5-alpha-reductase synthesis of DHT in the testes.
Testosterone Inhibitors ketoconazole aminoglutethimide	Inhibit adrenal synthesis of testosterone and other steroids.

DHT—dihydrotestosterone
LHRH—luteinizing hormone releasing hormone

is that the development of a refractory response by tumors can be delayed if different treatments are rotated.

This concludes the round-up of treatments typically employed against prostate cancer. The "cure" rate with any of these approaches for prostate cancer not confined to the prostate at diagnosis is below 20 percent.

There are three assumptions common to all of these forms of treatment. First, it is assumed that the cancer is a local phenomenon only—"really, the patient is completely healthy, he just happens to have prostate cancer." Second, it is assumed that testosterone and other androgens are the "enemy." Third, the treatment of the cancer and the current statistics on survival rates are almost always viewed in isolation. I ask you, what does it mean if the patient's prostate cancer was "cured," but he died of something else soon after?

My choice of therapy is integrative oncology, a fully balanced and complete approach to cancer, which is not built upon the foregoing assumptions.

Something New: Integrative Oncology

First, let's agree that no man exists in a void, but lives in direct relationship with his environment. We know that there are not only cancer-causing agents, such as various insecticides and PCBs, but also cancer-inducing situations and cancer-prone personalities. The goal should be to improve the quality of life for the patient, his family, and his friends, and not merely the length of life for the sake of statistics.

Second, life is all about change and dynamic balance. From a medical perspective, this balance may be referred to as "health," the ability of the individual to retain his integrity and ability to respond to a constantly changing world. Disease, especially cancer, often is best viewed as "an adaptive response that has maladaptive consequences." This is one of the points that pioneering researchers such as Dr. Rudolph Steiner have attempted to clarify for us. Illnesses—in this case cancer—are actually displaced and often magnified bodily responses gone awry.

Illness can actually be viewed as a challenge to fully integrate the self, as well as an opportunity to take a step along one's personal path of growth and development. Those who triumphantly overcome cancer are not victims! It is within our power to revamp our eating habits, to become more physically active, to reduce our levels of stress, to resolve emotional conflicts—in short, to adopt new strategies for healthier living.

The key, however, is to know the real enemy and to then adopt the appropriate plan for response. There is an adage that says, "To discover a real problem is to find a real solution." Note the order here: Finding a real solution can only come *after* the discovery of the real problem. Do not assume that there is a one-size-fits-all approach to prostate cancer therapy.

Asking the Right Questions

When a man first comes to my clinic with prostate cancer, I ask myself, "Why did this man get this cancer at this time?" This question is important because I am looking at a particular person with his own individual physiology who has prostate cancer, and this cancer may have begun five or ten years before it actually manifested. I begin by treating the person, not the disease.

By asking more specific questions and discovering their answers, I am seeking a logical treatment plan. For example, I will ask, "What is the cancer trying to do?" Answers to this question can be found in the cytopathology report and will tell me exactly how aggressive the cancer is, as well as give insight into likely weaknesses in the patient, such as a defect in the p53 gene, which helps to prevent normal cells from turning cancerous.

If the patient has been treated previously, asking historical questions about the cancer's sensitivity to androgen blockade may provide an immediate avenue for slowing its growth and buying time. If the cancer is becoming less responsive to Lupron, for instance, then perhaps a triple drug blockade strategy will give us time to plan the next step. This drug therapy is not curative, to be sure. Nevertheless, if the cancer is really starting to grow and it has, until very recently, been controlled by an androgen blocker, then a triple cocktail may give us a temporary respite and time to regroup for a more serious counterattack.

I can ask other questions through blood tests. For example, why did the patient's immune system allow this cancer to grow? Was the immune system damaged by a B-cell (CMV) virus that is also acting as the prostate cancer promoter? If so, then a strategy to put the virus back in remission will be an important part of the treatment plan. Does the patient have a history of mononucleosis? Does he suffer from recurrent sore throats, swollen glands, generalized aches and fatigue? When was his last fever?

I ask these questions in part through blood tests. Is his B-cell count low? Are his NK cells fewer than they should be in the face of normal or elevated T-cell ratios? What are his viral titers (a measure of the total viral load found in the body)? Asking the relevant questions makes all the difference in the world.

Of course, one question leads to another, but then, treatment calls for a bit of detective work. If a virus didn't slow down the immune system, then we need to look elsewhere. What is the man's nutritional status? Is he deficient in nutrients such as viramin D, selenium, zinc, or vitamin C? Is he not eating properly, or is he not absorbing the nutrients from the food he eats? Two martinis and a burger with special sauce just don't cut it, and it is up to the doctor to ferret out this type of information.

Other questions reveal clues where they might least be expected. Where does the patient live? What does he do? What has he been exposed to that could have triggered the cancer? What are his hobbies? What, no hobbies? Wow! That's even worse!

There is no one right question we can ask. Each question reveals a fragment of the truth; each fragment is an important piece of the puzzle and a partial path toward treatment.

There really are no wrong questions, either. Any response that leads us to a dead end is one less path to explore. There are, of course, questions which lead us to reasonable treatment plans sooner rather than later, and these are born of experience and intuition. When you're dealing with cancer, anything that brings about the faster discovery of an effective treatment plan is good. Many of the most productive questions are detailed throughout this book and summarized in the algorithm charts in Appendix O for your physician to explore on your behalf.

To maximize the quality and quantity of your life is the best that I've ever been able to do for anyone, and with a little luck, we may see a "spontaneous remission." Questions in this arena ascend to musings about purpose, meaning, fulfillment and love. They are even harder to answer, as no blood test can help. They are *critical* questions because they often speak to the root of stress, and chronic stress suppresses the immune system.

Personalizing Diagnosis and Treatment

Several decades ago, Roger Williams of the University of Texas at Austin, one of the giants in the development of the field of nutrition, championed the idea of *biochemical individuality*. By this he meant that we are each genetically and biochemically unique and that even our seemingly fixed genetic propensities can be altered by nutrition and the environment. For instance:

- Some of us are better at detoxifying drugs and chemicals than are others.
- The diet that causes one person to lose weight may cause another to gain weight.
- Nutrient requirements, even among those who are closely related, may vary several-fold.
- Cancer genes respond to diet and environment in different ways in different individuals.

The awareness that a persons's nutrition and habits often need to be individualized to match their particular body chemistry has been extended in several ways since Roger Williams first presented his ideas in 1956. Significantly, one's blood type (O, A, B, AB) may influence how much, and of what types of, protein, carbohydrate, and fat can be safely eaten, whether exercise should be vigorously aerobic or muscle building or gentle and oriented toward stretching, how stress might best be released, and the diseases to which one is prone. Similarly, pharmacists have long known that different classes of drugs can have strikingly different effects in individuals drawn from different racial backgrounds.

If it is now well established that biochemical individuality is an important variable in human health and disease, then it might well be asked why it plays such a small or even nonexistent role in therapies for prostate cancer. Good question. You'll find answers regarding specialized blood and urine tests, individualized programs for nutrition and detoxification, and suggestions for herbal and other supplements in the following chapters.

Restoring Balance: The Immune System and Endocrine Support

Individuals with cancer almost always have imbalances in two of the body's primary systems, the immune system and the endocrine system. These systems are closely intertwined, and therefore both must be balanced.

The immune system is the defensive army that the body uses to protect itself against infection. It defends against the daily attacks of bacteria, viruses, fungi, parasites, and cancer cells. This task requires a major commitment of the body's total resources. Yet the role of the immune system does not end with its defense against external invaders. The immune system also protects against the damage caused by exposure to ultraviolet rays and radioactivity, removes worn out cells and scar tissue, and of course, acts as an internal policeman to guard us against the development of tumors. Why does one person catch a cold, but not another? What causes allergies? How does cancer develop? In all of these cases, look to the immune system for the answers.

Good health depends largely upon making the immune system more active. If you want to improve your health, you need to stimulate immune function.

Occasionally, however, the immune system can become "overactive" instead of "underactive." On the one hand, the immune system needs vigilante macrophages, natural killer cells, and other "soldiers" to be on alert to attack invading organisms, such as the cold virus, before these can take hold in the body.

On the other hand, rheumatoid arthritis and other autoimmune diseases in which the body attacks itself afflict millions of Americans. "Overactivity" of certain components of the immune system can cause unpleasant side effects, such as allergies and inflammation, and can lead to immune exhaustion and collapse. In reality it is an underactivity of the T8 cytostatic (suppressor) cells that can lead to these autoimmune diseases. *Balance is the key!*

Immune overactivity such as allergies, and its subsequent exhaustion, may play a major role in the failure to eliminate cancerous cells in the early stages of tumor development. Immune "overactivity" is a prime source of free radicals in the body, as well as a drain upon the body's reserves of antioxidants. Free radicals are known initiators of cancers, and if the glutathione antioxidant system fails in prostate cells, they may become cancerous.

Closely linked to immune function is the endocrine system, the system of glands that secrete hormones such as adrenaline into the bloodstream. Modern living habits are sometimes said to "crank up" the "fight or flight" responses of the body, responses that originally had great value in assuring our survival many millennia ago. However, under modern conditions of limited physical activity and restraints upon the acting out of aggressive and fearful impulses, it is as if the body turns upon itself. Other emotions are tied into the endocrine and immune systems.

On the one hand, feelings of love, gratitude, and altruism improve immune response. The heart, which is not normally considered an endocrine gland, apparently secretes healing substances in response to positive emotions. On the other hand, depression, guilt, poor self-esteem, and apathy strongly depress the immune response. Major illnesses follow with distressing regularity upon the heels of depression and apathy after a divorce or the death of a loved one.

Fortunately, a great deal can be done about imbalances in both the immune and the endocrine systems. In my experience, detoxification, immunomodulation, endocrine regulation, and general nutritional support, if properly integrated into a program matched to the actual condition of the individual, can dramatically alter the odds in favor of successfully winning the battle against prostate cancer. Fortunately, in recent years the arsenal of weapons available for this fight has increased greatly. Many of these items, which I use, have few (if any) side effects in comparison with standard drug regimens, and they bring unusual benefits. Following are some of the categories of benefits found with alternative treatments. Please note that some products, such as PC SPES, are actually mixtures of several herbs, and these constituent herbs generally are discussed under that title rather than separately.

NEW THERAPIES

Antiandrogen-like Effects—PC SPES®.

Immune Activators—Natural killer cell support complex, Kinetrex®, and various mushroom and herbal products.

Immunomodulators and Supporters—AIDBCWE, vitamin C, flower pollen extracts, plant sterols and sterolins, licorice extracts.

Inducers of Cancer Cell Apoptosis (programmed cell death)—Urtica extract complex, PC SPES®, pollen extracts.

Glutathione Regulators—Glutathione precursors, such as ALA, N-acetyl-cysteine.

Detoxification Adjuncts—Herbal liver and colon detoxifiers, potassium, iodine/herbal complex, Calcium D-Glucarate, D-limonene, urtica extract complex, antioxidant formula, methyl donors (including s-adenosyl-methionine and trimethylglycine).

Inhibitors of Adhesion of Cancer Cells to Normal Tissues—Omega 3, 6, and 9 fatty acids, shark liver oil, modified citrus pectin, chondroitin sulfates.

CHAPTER FOUR

The Promise of PC SPES

An informed patient is also called a survivor.
A highly informed patient is referred to as a long-term survivor.

PC-SPES offers hope to thousands of prostate cancer victims, extending their lives while the battle to find a cure rages on.

—James Lewis, Jr., Ph.D.

Case Study: Tim J. is a 71-year-old gentleman with a 9-year history of prostate cancer that was originally treated with a prostatectomy and radiation therapy. Seven years ago, he began androgen blockade. Except for the side effects, this served him well until two years ago when the cancer recurred and spread. He began looking into alternative therapies, but these were only partially helpful. Fourteen months ago, when his PSA was at 87, he began an integrative treatment protocol. It began with a six-month break from any hormonal manipulation, during which time he received nutritional IVs, IV Iscucin, Beta-1,3-Glucan, and several supplements including vitamin C, AIDBCWE, antioxidants, food state multivitamin/mineral, CoQ-10, selenium, and niacin. Then he was given PC SPES, shark liver oil, flaxseed oil, and vitamin E. He was also changed to subcutaneous injections of Iscucin. With his PSA now at 0.8 and his liver and bone enzymes normal, he reports feeling "very well." His only complaint is his golf swing.

Commentary: If prostate cancer is detected at a very early stage, it can be "cured" in many men through the radical measures discussed earlier. Often, however, this "cure" does not hold and the cancer reappears several years later. Moreover, most men discover their prostate cancer when radical intervention is too late too improve either the length or the quality of life. In the majority of cases, the cancer is detected after it has spread. Palliative treatments, such as combination hormone therapy (CHT), typically buy time, but usually begin to fail a few years later when the cancer becomes refractory. Perhaps as bad as the poor rate of long-term success is the fact that most of the available treatments do little to improve or even maintain the quality of life.

The standard therapy for prostate cancer is to deprive the cancerous cells of certain hormones (usually considered to be the androgens or "male" hormones) that appear to fuel the cancer cells' growth. This approach is commonly termed "combination hormone blockade" (CHB) or "total androgen blockade" (TAB). CHB is not generally considered to be a cure, yet it does control prostate cancer growth to the point that the cancer is no longer a threat to the man's life in a significant percentage of patients, at least for a short period of time. Unfortunately, prostate cancer eventually becomes resistant to primary androgen blockade treatment. Although effective treatment protocols are available for patients with progressive cancer via CHB, this effectiveness is generally not of lasting duration.

The realization that CHB, TAB, and similar regimens eventually fail has given rise to the search for alternatives, and some of these alternative/complementary therapies already have borne fruit. PC SPES is perhaps the most promising of these recent alternative therapies. To date, there have been three reported clinical trials with PC SPES. The generally agreed upon findings are that, at least in the short term, PC SPES can have a *dramatic* effect upon PSA levels. Also reported are significant improvements in the quality of life, increases in energy levels and decreases in pain levels. In test tube cell cultures, PC SPES causes the death of certain lines of prostate cancer cells. However, there is no direct evidence yet of this in animal or clinical studies, albeit some physician researchers feel that the compound may exercise some true anticancer actions.

I am not proposing that PC SPES is a "magic bullet" for prostate cancer, but it is a valuable complement to other treatment protocols, and is a powerful armament in the new arsenal of complementary and alternative therapies. The trick is to match the right therapy to the individual and to rotate to a new therapy when a previously successful therapy begins to fail. This is what integrative oncology is all about. If what you're doing isn't working, find out why and do something else. Integrative oncology provides lots of treatment options centered around you as an individual.

The first step in my protocol is to use PC SPES to dramatically reduce PSA levels and enhance the quality of life. Nevertheless, this is only the first step. Cancer always denotes systemic problems in the body, and no localized treatment, no matter how good, will be permanent if the factors that contributed to the cancer are not addressed. The second step in my approach is to detoxify the body, to make changes in the diet and habits and in other ways, to correct the causative elements. The third step in my program is to reactivate the immune system. Cancers develop only when the immune system fails to properly police the body. PC SPES may not be a magic bullet, but it is the first of three essential steps on the way to controlling prostate cancer.

Another physician with considerable experience with PC SPES is Dr. Aaron Katz, Assistant Professor of Urology at Columbia Presbyterian Hospital in New York. Dr. Katz has given his views in several different forums on PC SPES, in light of his own clinical experiences. He is also a proponent of intermittent hormone therapy (IHT, described earlier) because he feels it both lowers the cost of the treatment (he typically uses a combination of Lupron and Zoladex) and extends the time before a patient begins to resist hormone treatment. He uses PC SPES as an adjunct to hormonal therapy rather than as a replacement after hormonal therapy has failed.

This is the way I begin my therapeutic strategy:

If a man comes to me on hormonal blockade drug therapy, and it is working for him, then I will usually switch him to an intermittent dosing of the triple drug blockade that I like, start him on PC SPES, even if it makes the side effects of the drugs a bit worse, and use the time that the drugs are buying us to work on jump-starting his immune system. During the times that he is off of the drugs, I still keep him on the PC SPES as it increases the time before I would restart the drugs and thus decreases the side effects that he may experience overall. In this particular approach, PC SPES is used as an assist to hormonal therapy rather than as a replacement after hormonal therapy has failed.

However, I have noticed that among my patients who have failed conventional antiandrogen therapy, many eventually become resistant to the good effects of PC SPES as well. When this happens, the PSA scores begin to rise as the cancer again takes hold. Thus, a patient needs an extended treatment program using my immunotherapy strategies to prevent or minimize the possibility of a relapse even when PC SPES is being employed as a treatment.

Ideally, one should start the PC SPES *before* taking the antiandrogen drugs because the overall response is much better with far fewer side effects and a lower dose of the PC SPES. To date, I have not seen any men who began therapy with PC SPES—instead of drugs—become refractory! However, due to its side effects, some men have had to go off PC SPES. Thanks to P-Care®, this is changing.

PC SPES is an important component of my first line of therapy since it seems to have direct anticancer effects. A number of physicians who are employing PC SPES have come to similar conclusions. Let's look again at the practice of Dr. Aaron Katz. He used PC SPES in a program for 80 patients, 15 of whom had failed with various previous therapies. Under Katz's protocol, standard hormonal therapy was used for roughly seven months to reduce PSA readings to acceptable levels. At this point, hormonal treatment was discontinued and the patients began 3 capsules of PC SPES per day. Those who were hormonally refractory were started on 6 capsules per day. All patients were tested for PSA bimonthly. As long as the patient's PSA levels remain stable, the program is continued. Although Dr. Katz has not published any long-term data, his results at six months with 49 of these patients showed that PSA levels were still declining in this group. This reflects my experience of over four years, and most of my PC SPES patients are still going strong!

Typical side effects when using PC SPES by itself are nipple tenderness and breast enlargement in about 90 percent of cases, and most men will experience a marked decline in libido. Many men will find that some aspects of their mood are tied to their libido, of course. There are reports of other symptoms that may be related to

PC SPES, as well: diarrhea in 5 percent of cases, calf pains in 3 to 5 percent, and blood clots in 3 to 5 percent of cases *may* also be related to it. Curiously these side effects are similar to those found by patients taking diethylstilbestrol (DES). To protect against blood clots, I advise patients to take daily: an aspirin, 400 IU of vitamin E, garlic tablets, fish oil, vitamin A and flaxseed oil. Others have found that a largely vegetarian diet with many soy-based products (fermented soy liquid drinks are especially effective) reduces nipple tenderness; other estrogen-like side effects can be helped with urtica extract complex.

Patients who are most successful in using PC SPES for two years and more, without immune support, seem to be men who concurrently take finasteride, urtica extract complex, or another substance that blocks the transformation of testosterone to dihydrotestosterone (DHT). PC SPES has a number of estrogen-like actions, which can have powerful and contradictory effects upon a man's body. On the positive side, pharmaceutical estrogen therapy suppresses the production of testosterone by affecting the pituitary gland, and large amounts of estrogen will reduce the binding of testosterone to cell receptors by competing for those receptor sites. There is even some evidence that estrogens may be directly toxic to prostate cancer tumors, at least in the short run.

On the other hand, however, estrogens also reduce the body's clearance of DHT from prostate cells and appear to magnify DHT's impact in both prostate cancer and BPH. Inhibiting estrogen's impact upon DHT binding by reducing overall levels of DHT would seem to be a good adjunctive therapy. Although drugs that inhibit the conversion of testosterone to DHT (such as finasteride) have not proven to be of great benefit against prostate cancer when used alone, trials have shown considerable positive effects when a DHT inhibitor is added to hormone treatments to reduce testosterone levels and, as a result, increase estrogen levels in the body. This should be kept in mind when using PC SPES, and it is a very good reason to use supplements like P-Care® and flaxseed oil.

I have had very good success in my practice using PC SPES as part of my broader approach. I have yet to determine whether PC SPES will continue to maintain low PSA levels for three or more years for a significant number of men with prostate cancer without being matched with the other measures I use in my practice. I am thus cautioning against using PC SPES by itself as yet another "magic bullet" against cancer. However, even skeptics must admit that PC SPES has proven itself useful for many patients who have already failed with other treatments, and that the side effects are less serious than with Lupron/Casodex™ and related therapies. PC SPES is thus an important and powerful part of an integrated treatment protocol.

What Is PC SPES?

The story of PC SPES, as it is usually told, starts with chemist Sophie Chen, Ph.D., and Allan Wang, M.D. These two first collaborated in 1986 to create a new cancer treatment based upon the herbal knowledge inherited from Dr. Wang's family and the knowledge of modern biotechnology brought by Dr. Chen. The first result was a formula, which when tested in Chinese hospitals, showed real promise for reducing the pain and debilitation associated with cancer. The product was named SPES to signify "hope" (from the Latin *spes*).

The current PC SPES formula is a refinement of that earlier research. Named PC SPES only in 1996 to indicate hope for prostate cancer, the formula actually was developed in 1990 for a Taiwanese relative of Dr. Chen who had been diagnosed with terminal prostate cancer. After five years of using PC SPES, Dr. Chen's relative remained symptom-free with a PSA reading of less than 1 ng/ml. At first, PS SPES was produced almost entirely for research purposes. However, in 1994 the formula had become well enough known for a demand to develop for it in the United States.

The eight herbs used in PC SPES have been shown to exhibit anti-tumor, antiviral, and immune-stimulating properties. All are traditional Chinese herbs except for the American plant *Serenoa repens* (saw palmetto), which is now widely recognized to aid in reducing prostate enlargement and inflammation (See *Saw Palmetto for Men and Women* by David Winston). Painstaking quality control is practiced to ensure that the individual extracts remain consistent from batch to batch and that the entire mixture works together synergistically.

TEN PROPOSED BIOLOGICAL ACTIONS OF PC SPES

1. Suppresses prostate cancer cell growth.
2. Reduces intracellular PSA.
3. Reduces secreted PSA.
4. Decreases the quantity of prostate cell androgen receptors.
5. Decreases the affinity of androgen binding to androgen receptor sites.
6. Decreases clonogenicity (ability of cancer cells to develop colonies).
7. Slows the tumor cell growth cycle and decreases cell replication.
8. Causes apoptosis (programmed cell death).
9. Suppresses the apoptosis-resistance protein (the bcl-2 protein).
10. Enhances tumor radiation sensitivity.

PC SPES—A Vital Step to an Integrated Approach

The usual approach to treating prostate cancer is to treat the cancer, not the patient. PC SPES is different. The eight herbs have multiple effects that make this compound suitable to individuals whose health and basic constitutions vary widely. For instance, by acting as an antiviral, PC SPES may help to partially relieve the burden on the immune system. Its direct antitumor properties are complemented by its ability to stimulate the immune system. PC SPES also has anti-inflammatory benefits, and these, again, support immune function and may help to inhibit one of the ways in which cancers spread and metastasize. Moreover, its actions against benign hyperplasia may serve to improve the quality of life, even aside from its effects upon the prostate cancer itself and is another indication for its use that I employ in my practice.

Let's take a look at the individual herbs found in this formula and then at some of the theories as to how the product works. The makers of PC SPES maintain that only certified organic herbs are used for production. This means that they do not need to contend with problems of contamination with environmental toxins. It also means that the "profile" of constituents of the herbs will not have been altered by the use of modern fertilizers that act as xenoestrogens and aggravate prostate cancer. Once harvested, the herbs are extracted and standardized according to proprietary methods.

Here are the common names of each herb used in this compound, followed by the scientific name and one of the forms of Romanized Chinese names. Saw palmetto is a Western herb and thus does not have a Chinese name.

*Chrysanthemum (*Dendranthema morifolium *Tzvel, Chu-hua)*

Traditionally used in Chinese medicine for these properties and/or against these conditions: "sedative; refigerant in headache; influenza; purgative; antitoxic." Translated into English, Western medicine would say that it is an anti-inflammatory with some immune-regulating properties.

*Isatis (*Isatis indigotica *Fort, Ta-ching-yeh)*

Traditionally used in Chinese medicine for these properties and/or against these conditions: "cools blood; removes toxins; cleanses and soothes throat." Western research has focused upon its constituents called phytosterols (plant sterols), items that are similar in structure to cholesterol and that often help to regulate human responses to hormones, such as estrogens. Beta-sitosterol is a common sterol in Isatis. Under some conditions, this compound has been shown experimentally to reduce tumor growth in animals.

*Licorice (*Glycyrrhiza glabra *L., Gan-cao)*

Traditionally used in Chinese medicine for these properties and/or against these conditions: "anti-inflammatory for arthritis or allergic conditions; digestive stimulant; lung disorders." Licorice spares the adrenal glands by reducing the demand upon them to produce corticosteroids. It is useful against some liver disorders and improves the production of bile. It is useful against some cancers, including hepatic cancer. More especially, licorice reduces the debilitating effects of many poisons and toxins.

*Ganoderma (*Ganoderma lucidum *Karst, Ling-zhi)*

Traditionally used in Chinese medicine for these properties and/or against these conditions: "immune stimulant; anti-bacterial; anti-allergenic; anti-inflammatory; anti-tussive." One of the most prized of Chinese herbs, this mushroom has been shown to be a powerful anticancer agent.

*Pseudo-ginseng or Notoginseng (*Panax pseudo-ginseng *Wall, San-chi)*

Traditionally used in Chinese medicine for these properties and/or against these conditions: "analgesic; stops internal and external bleeding." This herb has demonstrated antiviral and antibacterial effects as well as influencing the actions of the liver. It reduces capillary permeability; this property might reduce the impact of inflammation upon tissues. Some authors have suggested that it may increase natural killer (NK) cell activity.

*Rubescens (*Rabdosia rubescens, *Don-ling-cao)*

Traditionally used in Chinese medicine for these properties and/or against these conditions: "tumors; cancer; arthralgia; headaches." In *in vitro* tests, the extract has been shown to inhibit the growth of a large variety of cancers. Antineoplastic effects have been observed in human patients. Furthermore, the herb has been observed to reduce weight loss and to increase survival time in cancer patients.

*Saw Palmetto (*Serenoa repens*)*

In Western experience, saw palmetto is useful as an antiseptic diuretic that reduces benign prostate enlargement.

*Scute (*Scutellaria baicalensis *Georgi, Huang-chin)*

Traditionally used in Chinese medicine for these properties and/or against these conditions: "removes toxins; gastroenteritis; water retention." In quite a number of *in vitro* experiments, scute has been found to inhibit cancer cell growth and even to induce in cancer cells *apoptosis*, or cell death. It improves immune function and possesses wide-ranging antiviral and antibacterial properties.

Success in Unpromising Cases

Even though I have been using PC SPES for over four years, it is still considered an "alternative" treatment for prostate cancer, and is not well known. Now—finally—research studies are coming out that mirror my clinical experience and success with PC SPES. In 1999, Dr. Eric Small and his colleagues at the University of California at San Francisco reported results from an ongoing two-year study of PC SPES in 61 cancer patients, ages 43 to 90. The preliminary findings were released in Atlanta at the 35th annual meeting of the American Society of Clinical Oncology and were widely reported. Thirty-four of the patients in the report were men whose cancers were no longer responding to standard hormonal treatments (hormonally refractive cases) and the other 27 were men who had not been treated with hormones ("hormonal virgins") and thus still had largely androgen-dependent cancers. By the third week of the study, all the subjects were taking three capsules (960 milligrams) of PC SPES three times per day.

The benefits of this protocol clearly appeared in several cases that Dr. Small handled. PSA levels were initially quite high in all the men in the study. In the 27 patients who previously had not received hormone treatments, 56 percent experienced drops in their PSA to *undetectable levels*, and levels dropped by at least *50 percent* in the remaining members of this group! Quite remarkably, in 19 of the 34 men with hormonally refractive cancers, the PSA levels dropped by *more* than 50 percent! Nearly one half of the men in the latter group had also undergone second-line hormone treatment.

Transrectal ultrasound tests confirmed these benefits in men who had not previously been treated with hormones. In 50 percent of the 16 men tested from the hormone-naive group (that is, those with mostly androgen-dependent tumors), there was a reduction of more than 50 percent in tumor volume. In the other group of men whose cancers were androgen-independent, 22 were known to have metastases to the bones. Only 12 of these men were available for retesting in time for the release of results in Atlanta, and of these, 2 had experienced dramatic improvements since beginning treatment with PC SPES.

On the other hand, Dr. Small found that almost all his patients on PC SPES had reduced levels of testosterone (81%) and experienced gynecomastia (nipple tenderness and enlargement, 92%), which can be helped with other supplements. PC SPES thus has powerful estrogenic effects. In a later chapter, I will discuss the use of several supplements such as flaxseed oil to reduce these estrogen-like side effects.

In a 1999 seminar on prostate cancer, Dr. Small revealed to his audience that PC SPES appeared to have anticancer properties. Now other researchers are testing PC SPES. In San Diego, Dr. Israel Barken is overseeing another trial, also involving 25 patients. Dr. Charles Myers is conducting trials at the University of Virginia. Not yet available are the results of a trial involving 25 patients conducted by Dr. Abraham Mittleman of New York Medical College. In preliminary reports based upon only 15 patients, Dr. Mittleman indicated that the quality of life of those taking PC SPES improved (better appetite, greater energy, less pain, and a generally greater feeling of well-being) and that in at least one patient, the PSA level had declined from 180 to 0.80 in four and one-half years. In another, the PSA had declined from 150 to 9 in twelve months. These trials should begin to answer such questions as whether PC SPES should be used in conjunction with or, perhaps in advance of, treatments that weaken immune response, how long the results from PC SPES hold up before patients again become refractory, and so forth.

Zbigniew Darzynkiewicz, M.D., Ph.D., and National Institutes of Health Merit Fellow, has been very active in investigating the mechanisms of action of PC SPES. At the Cancer Research Institute of New York Medical College, my alma mater, he found that PC SPES can kill a number of lines of cancer cells, including prostate cancer. Significantly, the levels of the extracts that were effective *in vitro* should be possible to achieve *in vivo*, including in human patients. The work of Dr. Darzynkiewicz and other researchers has indicated, in particular, that PC SPES may reduce the expression of the gene bcl-2, a gene that is active in cancer cells. Suppressing this gene may be one avenue by which PC SPES causes apoptosis. In other words, PC SPES may work, in part, by activating the preprogrammed death of cancer cells!

PC SPES also may influence the growth cycle of cancer cells so as to directly slow their growth. It suppresses androgen receptors and has strong estrogenic-like actions, although these effects presently have not been explained in terms of the traditional herbs used. However, it is quite clear that even from the usual descriptions of these extracts, PC SPES derives a synergistic effect from its eight herbs. The company marketing PC SPES offers the following summary of benefits by category:

PUBLICATIONS ON PC SPES

1. Antitumor activity
   A. Ganoderma lucidum Karst: Maruyama *et al., J. Pharmacobiodyn*, 1989, Feb.12(2):118–23.
   B. Rabdosia rubescens: Wang *et al., Chung Hun-Chung-Liu-Tsa-Chih* 1986 Jul; 8(4):297–99.
   C. Scutellaria baicalensis Georgi: Konoshitna *et al., Chem Phar. Bull.* Tokyo 1992, Feb. 40(2):531–33.
2. Immune-stimulating activity
   A. Ganoderma lucidum Karst: Ed. New Medical College of Jian-Su Province, *Encyclopedia of Chinese Medicinal Herbs*, 1975, pp. 2395–99, by Shanghai People's Publisher.
   B. Isatis indigotica Fort: Xu *et al., Chung-Hsi-I-Chieh-Ho-Tsa-Chin* 1991, June 11 (6):357–59, 3225–26.
3. Antiviral activity
   A. Scutelleria baicalensis Georgi: Nagai *et al., Biol. Pharm. Bull.* 1995, Feb. 18(2):285–89. Li *et al., Cell Mol. Biol. Res.* 1993.39:(22):1 19–24.
   B. Dendranthema (Chrysanthemum) morifolium Tzvel: He *et al., J. Natural Products*, 1994 Jan. 57(1):42–51.
4. Anti-inflammatory activity
   A. Scutellaria baicalensis Georgi: Butenko *et al., Agents Actions*, 1993, 39 Spec. No.: 49–51.
   B. Glycyrrhiza glabra L.: Kobayashis *et al., Biol. Pharm. Bull.* 1995 Oct. 18 (10):1382–85.
5. Anti-benign prostate hyperplasia activity
   Serena repens: Dralkorn *et al., Urologe* A., 1995. 34(2):119–29.

More Promises on the Horizon

PC SPES represents but one example of what can be achieved against prostate cancer through a carefully integrated approach on an herbal level. The cancer is attacked simultaneously on several fronts, and at the same time, the body is supported in one or more of its major systems. The outcome is called "synergism," and is much more powerful: the whole result is greater than the sum of the parts.

As we'll see in the next chapter, the arsenal available for the battle against prostate cancer has many more weapons in it than you may have guessed. For instance, special extracts made from flower pollen have been shown to cause apoptosis of prostate cancer cell lines when tested in much the same fashion as has been done with PC SPES. Flower pollen extracts, like several of the herbs found in PC SPES, can boost the immune system, reduce inflammation, and fight BPH. Natural compounds similar in action to the drug finasteride can reduce the conversion of testosterone to dihydrotestosterone; other compounds can support and regulate endocrine function, etc.

In the next chapter, you'll follow one man's journey as he fights prostate cancer and discovers that life can still be quite rewarding in spite of the cancer.

CHAPTER FIVE

When the Other Guy Is You—
One Man's Journey

Diseases only attack those whose outer circumstances, particularly food, are faulty. . . . The prevention and banishment of disease are primarily matters of food; secondarily, of suitable conditions of environment. Antiseptics, medicaments, inoculations, and extirpating operations evade the real problem. Disease is the censor pointing out the humans, animals and plants who are imperfectly nourished.

—G. T. Wrench, *The Wheel of Health*

Entering a New World

Hi. I'm Lee Heiman, an editor at Kensington Publishing. Jesse Stoff is my doctor and he asked me to write a chapter for this book from the point of view of the patient. You see, like many of you who are reading this volume, *I have prostate cancer.*

I never expected to develop cancer. What man does? Of course, I expected that as I got older my body would start to show the wear and tear of age, but I was prepared for a little arthritis, not cancer. Like most other men, I never thought of myself as being vulnerable to a potentially fatal sickness or disease. I had denial down pat. You know:

"It will go away."
"It will stop on its own."
"Whatever it is, I can 'learn to live with it.' "

Cancer, I learned, isn't something you "learn to live with." It changes your life, and after more than 60 years, I was not prepared for this type of change. Let's face it for most of us life is a routine—

usually a comfortable one. We have the foods we like, the diversions we enjoy, our hopes that the next day will be better than the last. And naturally, there are the annoyances and stress we never seem to be able to overcome, plus our ways of "letting off steam"—strategies often as unhealthful as the stresses they are meant to overcome. But through it all, we expect that our bodies will just keep chugging along, that nothing fundamental will go wrong despite the fact that we usually take better care of our pets and our cars than we do ourselves. When something bad does happen, we're surprised, if not shocked.

When I was diagnosed with prostate cancer, I was stunned. I had always been in relatively good health. Yes, I was a little too intense, a bit too consumed with my projects and inclined to bring work home. I might have expected an ulcer, but I never made the connection between stress and cancer. Looking back on things now, I can hardly believe how many of the foods and habits I took for granted are truly health damaging. Cancer gave me a wake-up call.

Perhaps there had been small signs for a long time that things weren't as they should be with my body but I had ignored the symptoms. However, in late October, 1998, something happened I could not ignore.

I was returning to the office after seeing a client in New York City when I began to feel a sudden urgency to find a men's room. I had had a little more coffee than usual that morning, so I thought nothing of this urgency—at first. I entered my building and frantically rushed to the elevator hoping to make it to the men's room.

Surprise! I was still in the elevator when I felt a warm sensation trickle down my leg. I had lost bladder control!

Yet as upset as I was, I quickly began making excuses. "I am 67 and getting old . . . stuff happens . . . I just waited too long. . . ." I knew that something was wrong, but never suspected cancer. Perhaps I just found ways not to go in that direction.

However, I did contact my son-in-law, a pediatrician, who arranged for me to see a urologist in the New York City area. I'll call him Dr. A. Dr. A gave me a blood test called the prostate specific antigen test (PSA for short). On November 15, 1998, the results came back high—and they weren't good. "Normal" readings are between 0 and 4 in my age group. My score was 15.7. As Jesse already discussed earlier, the PSA test, as is true of many medical tests, can give unusual results for more than one reason. Dr. A suggested that a possible infection in my prostate gland could have raised my PSA levels and given a false reading. I was put on antibiotics for two weeks and then the test was repeated.

Unfortunately, the result from the repeat test was not what I was hoping for. Rather than going down, my score the second time around was even higher at 15.9. With such an elevated PSA score, the most likely diagnosis is prostate cancer, and Dr. A wanted to immediately perform a biopsy to collect tissue samples from my prostate and have these checked for cancerous cells. I refused, having heard that the biopsy might actually spread the cancer if it was present or might even cause cancer if it wasn't already there.

A few weeks later, I went to a second doctor for another opinion. Dr. B arranged for PSA tests at his own laboratory, and found that my PSA score was only 3.6 and that my free PSA, a more sophisticated measure, was a reassuring 100 percent. The second opinion was that I did not have cancer.

Now, I was both relieved and confused. Which lab was correct? I, of course, preferred to believe that Dr. B had the right of things.

So I got a third opinion. I set up an appointment for yet another PSA test at New York's Columbia Presbyterian Hospital. The results came back on February 8, 1999. They were even higher—19.9. More tests results from Dr. A arrived at about the same time. These were 22.3. My original alarm was giving way to outright panic.

In case any reader should get the feeling that my concerns were just about numbers, let me set the record straight. My ability to control my urination had deteriorated to the point that I planned out my work day around access to a men's room. If I went anywhere in the city, I always knew exactly where the rest rooms were. And at home I had to run water in the sink in order to relax enough to urinate. I actually found myself counting the seconds that I had a urine stream! Fifteen seconds was too short, but if I could just keep the stream going for. . . .

Beyond Denial

Somewhat like a medieval pilgrim journeying from holy place to holy place seeking a cure, I began visiting famous medical institutions around the country, hoping someone would tell me this was all a bad dream. Sloan Kettering Hospital in New York performed a PSA test in mid-April that registered a reading of 7.37, although the physician at that institute thought this score clearly warranted a biopsy. Again, I refused. A test performed in California yielded a score of 21.6 at about the same time. Finally, yet another test at Sloan Kettering in the first week of May indicated a PSA of 39.1 with a free PSA of 14.9. A PSA of 39.1 is a seriously elevated score, which indicates not just the presence of prostate cancer, but of cancer that has almost certainly spread outside of the prostate.

Now, I was really alarmed. When my PSA score was only 15—I can hardly believe that I now can say "only" and "15" in the same breath—it was possible to hold on to the belief that something other than cancer was involved.

At this point it was obvious that Dr. B had been wrong and that the original test performed by Dr. A had been correct all along. Yet, it appeared I was being diagnosed with cancer, and I wouldn't accept this diagnosis without a fight.

Another pilgrimage took me to the medical school at the University of California at San Francisco. There, a special type of scan called spectroscopy on April 27 showed prostate cancer. It had spread throughout the entire prostate to the seminal ducts, to part of the hip bone and to the pubic bone. Subsequent tests, including a biopsy and a bone scan confirmed that all lobes of the prostate were involved and that the cancer had spread into the surrounding tissues. My Gleason Score, 8 out of 10, was extremely high and indicated a quite virulent cancer.

What's that saying: "You can run, but you can't hide." Friends and relatives die, we see and hear about cancer and other illnesses all the time, yet somehow it isn't truly real until something happens to us personally. Until cancer happens to us personally, it always happens to the "other guy." Then, all at once, *we* have become the "other guy."

New Hope With PC SPES

Fortunately I had been working with Dr. Jesse Stoff of Arizona on a book about prostate cancer. Dr. Stoff used the herbal compound PC SPES in his practice with his prostate cancer patients.

After consultations with Dr. Stoff, I decided to try PC SPES on my own. It was available without prescription, as it is an herbal product. I started taking it on May 24 at the rate of nine capsules per day (three capsules three times per day). I also began a supplement and food modification program. Thus far all my news had gone from bad to worse. So I wasn't too hopeful when I returned one month later for yet another PSA test. This time, however, things were different.

June 12—My PSA score was 3.1.
June 24—PSA score was 1.3.
June 29—PSA score is 0.9
September 9—PSA score is 0.35 when taken at Dr. Stoff's office!

This dramatic fall in my PSA scores is impressive even when compared with the pretty radical improvements many patients see when they start using PC SPES. A big part of my success came not just from the herbal compound, but also from the fact that, at Dr. Stoff's suggestion, I began to implement changes in my diet at the same time that I began to use the PC SPES.

Jesse Stoff to the Rescue

In order to appreciate just what a difference a few months meant to me, you have to look beyond the PSA scores. The falling PSA scores supplied a spark of hope in an otherwise relentlessly grim picture.

Even before Jesse and I had met for the first time, we had talked about working on this book. I had formed some impression of him, but nothing had prepared me for my first office visit.

Jesse was one big surprise package. He's a jovial fellow who likes to greet patients with a vigorous welcome and a big hug. No cold clinician, Jesse is open, friendly, and loving, and he makes this openness and good cheer an important part of his practice.

Unlike most of the other doctors who had seen my statistics, Jesse definitely was *not* the incarnation of the Grim Reaper. For instance, when asked regarding my high PSA scores, his response was, "Don't worry, I've seen a lot worse, even patients who had scores in the thousands! PSA and Gleason scores are, after all, just numbers!" After months of getting medical opinion after opinion, each more pessimistic than the last, Jesse's optimism was uplifting.

Following my check-up and the taking of a "history" to learn what was happening in my life, I was ushered into the presence of the in-house acupuncturist and specialist in Chinese diagnostics and herbs. My tongue was checked, then multiple pulses were taken. I was told that my kidneys—the seat of vital energy in Chinese diagnostics—were weak. An herbal tea was prescribed to strengthen the kidneys and the liver. I also had a session with acupuncture needles to strengthen my immune response.

Next was a massage. That's right, a massage! As you can see, Jesse is not an ordinary physician. I had had a pain in my buttocks for weeks and had assumed that this pain was from a cancer site— which doctors had earlier agreed was the case. It was a constant reminder of my cancer and had begun to weigh heavily on me. Jesse quietly suggested that the pain could be coming from a muscle spasm. He was right! After my first massage, this pain went away!

It was amazing—I had been worrying and stressing over what had actually been a muscle strain. The renewed peace of mind from the removal of this pain was itself worth the office visit to me. But Jesse had more surprises in store. He uses meditation, guided imagery, and relaxation as part of his treatment.

Unlike the other doctors I had consulted, Jesse insisted that the mind-body connection be taken seriously. "If you want to survive, you've got to learn to relax," he told me. At the clinic, I even had a full psychological analysis performed by a professional psychologist. He pinpointed my emotional blockages and stress points. I have learned that there now is a whole subfield of medicine that studies the interaction of the immune system with neurological and emotional responses. I do feel better when I do the imagery and the relaxation exercises.

Jesse tailored my program to my individual needs. For instance, he noted that my blood type is B+, which suggests I should strictly limit my eating tomato products. On Jesse's advice, I also removed wheat, processed foods, caffeine, dairy and alcohol from my diet. Instead of sugar, I use Stevia, a natural sweetner. I added dark green vegetables, beets, salads, and green tea and I began to use supplements. I learned to enjoy "green drinks," such as those that contain dried barley juice. I lost 20 pounds I didn't need, and started to feel better.

Lee's Healing Program

Food

The start of my new food program was simplified by the food-state nutrients I was taking. The quote at the beginning of this chapter—"Diseases only attack those whose outer circumstances, particularly food, are faulty. The prevention and banishment of disease are primarily matters of food"—is so true. No one knows the exact structure of food. A simple tomato contains at least 10,000 phytonutrients (one of them being lycopene). Researchers are now saying a broad range of phytonutrients prevent and heal cancer. That's why I start my daily regimen with a supplement that contains 62 complex foods, herbs, vitamins, and minerals in the food state.

Learning which supplements to take and when was relatively easy to do. Adjusting my diet was much more difficult. Until I was diagnosed with cancer, I truly believed that my food intake was both healthy and nourishing. How little I knew! I didn't eat red meat often, kept away from fast-food restaurants, ate fish often—but I never passed up an offered cookie (or two), a slice of birthday cake, crackers with cheese, and so on. Soup and vegetables too often came from cans. All these foods are loaded with trans-fats, which Dr. Walter Willet of the Harvard School of Public Health has linked to the increase in prostate cancer. These foods also contain whopping amounts of sugar, chemicals, and salt.

Today, I eat virtually nothing that comes from a box, jar, can, or wrapper. The majority of my food has its origins, not in a processing plant, but directly from the earth and oceans. I now choose "power foods" loaded with nutrients for nourishment and healing. Here's my list.

Power Foods

1. Sweet potatoes or yams, beets, and squash. These I bake.
2. Whole grains—organic brown rice, whole oats, and occasionally some "ancient" grains, such as quinoa and spelt. I get my brown rice from a top-notch domestic farm, which also has delicious organic rice crackers and rice pasta.
3. Cruciferous vegetables such as broccoli, Brussels sprouts, and cabbage. These I lightly steam. If you oversteam these, you will lose enzymatic activity.
4. Dark leafy greans, which include kale, collards, and spinach, also cooked in my steamer. I also use beet greens from the top of the beets.
5. Onions, garlic, ginger, which I steam or enjoy raw. A very effective method to overcome the "smell" of garlic is to chew parsley sprinkled with lemon.
6. Raw salads (great for enzymes), which include romaine, radicchio, endive, and arugula. This is a great way to get enzymes into our bodies. Many studies indicate the need for enzymes, particularly as we age and/or illness overtakes us.
7. Mushrooms, particularly shitake, which I also steam. Additionally, there is a wonderful maitake solution I take with a dropper.
8. Raw carrots and red and green peppers are also part of my veggie regimen. I pack a small amount of these in a paper bag to take with me wherever I go.
9. Flaxseed. A wonderful source of omega-3. Use it sprinkled on other foods. (See also flax oil in the oil listings.)

Protein

Protein is a bit more difficult. All red meat is off limits when you have prostate cancer, but fish is not. I use salmon, canned sardines (my only exception to never using canned foods), grouper, tuna, and cod. I discovered a source for wild caught salmon (preferable to farm-raised) and other varieties of fish, which I've listed in the resource section.

I don't use chicken, but I love white meat from organic turkey, which you can get from your local health food store or from mail order sources. There is a lot of concern about eggs, but I'll have organic eggs approximately 1–2 times weekly. They're terrific complete protein.

I'll use beans to combine with my brown rice and other grains, and of course, soybeans. I love to steam whole soybeans that come in a frozen pack. They're tasty and nutritious. Tempeh, a fermented soy derivative, is a good source of protein. I'll steam it with my vegetables. I prefer this over tofu. I'm also very excited about a new fermented soy drink. Dr. Israel Barken offered details of a clinical study at the Third International Symposium on the Role of Soy in Preventing and Treating Chronic Disease in Washington, D.C., in November 1999. The study showed this drink could be a viable alternative to drugs, radiation, or surgery for prostate cancer patients, and slows the PSA rate.

Dr. Stoff is always concerned with all his prostate patients maintaining energy levels. His message is constant—"Get enough protein every day." A handful of raw almonds (keep refrigerated) on occasion is a great protein treat. And every couple of days, I'll use specially formulated whey protein powder, which I blend with water.

I try to avoid overly sweet fruits such as mangoes and watermelons. There is some question and controversy about the high sugar content being risky for prostate cancer.

But there is much to choose from among both winter and summer fruits. Apples are available almost all year and they're a favorite for me. I love bananas but will eat them only firm. When they're too soft, their glycemic index jumps. Tangerines and oranges are delicious and loaded with vitamin C. I eagerly purchase strawberries, blueberries, raspberries, and cherries whenever they're available at the store where I get my organic produce. I have a fondness for red grapes and, of course, kiwis.

Remember, adding more fresh organic fruits and vegetables is proably the most significant dietary change you can make, if you are truly interested in boosting and maintaining your wellness level.

Oils

Oils are a vital part of our daily diet. But which oils? Let's eliminate from consideration the heavily processed oils that can sit on supermarket shelves for long periods of time. Too often, they're loaded with trans-fats and chemicals, which absolutely can be dangerous.

1. High-lignan flax oil. Some people supplement with it directly from the bottle. I prefer to sprinkle it on other foods. Flax is a superb source for essential fatty acids, with an excellent ratio of omega-3 to omega-6 and 9. Never heat this oil, and keep it refrigerated at all times.

2. Extra virgin olive oil. In every study on the health benefits of the acclaimed Mediterrean diet, this is the oil of choice. I use it on every salad I eat. Keep it refrigerated.

3. My mother was right. Cod liver oil is a terrific source of valuable nutrients. I use a cod liver oil flavored with lemon. One teaspoon contains 2,000–2,500 IUs of vitamin A, 400–500 IUs of vitamin D, plus high levels of omega-3, including DHA, EPA and ALA. Refrigerate this oil.

4. There are some excellent fish oil supplements packaged in soft gels, for those who prefer not to have to taste fish oils.

I take a teaspoon of raw bee pollen every day. Some studies and anecdotal evidence show the pollen has provable restorative powers, and can perhaps help to shrink enlarged prostates It is also loaded with vitamins, enzymes, bioflavonoids, trace minerals, and carotenoids. Another gift from the bees is royal jelly, which is loaded with amino acids and nucleic acids (RNA and DNA), as well as beta-carotene and glutathione.

Fluids

Jesse advises juicing every day, using mostly greens. If I'm unable to juice every day, I've learned to improvise, using powdered green drinks, including a formula that contains a wide variety of greens, herbs, enzymes, mushrooms, and other power foods. Other powdered drinks I use are a potent green grasses and barley combo, as well as a wheat grass drink. I discovered delicious red beet formulas, which I'll use in the morning as well as for an afternoon pick up.

I also use noni juice, a rejuvenating, healthful drink that contains bromelaia, which seems to help my digestion.

No listing about food would be complete without water. Jesse recommends 8–9 glasses daily. Your body tissues require this much to function plus it acts as a great flush to wash away toxins.

I have discovered a special water which is twice purified to create a superpure water base. The source water is first purified through reverse osmosis and secondly purified with a proprietary process that further cleans the water of heavy metals and dissolved contaminants. From this base, a special formulation of minerals and electrolytes is added back to create a mild alkalinity with antioxidant properties (see Resource Section).

I sip water all day. As we age, and especially during the colder months, our bodies don't signal the need for water.

Don't forget green tea. This powerful antioxidant has proven effective against prostate cancer. I drink 3–5 cups every day. Green tea contains epigallocatechin-3-gallate, which has been shown to block the growth of, and shrink, human prostate cancers.

Condiments

I also have some healthy flavoring options. Sloan Kettering Hospital in NYC did studies showing that aged garlic extract has ingredients that act against prostate cancer. I found the product and use it on various foods every day. I also use cumin and tumeric, tasty and healthy spices.

Lest I forget, there are some terrific lines of tomato sauces and pastes. E. Giovannucci, M.D., of the Harvard University of Public Health in Boston, reported in studies that men who ate ten weekly servings of lycopene-rich tomato sauces were 45 percent less likely to develop prostate cancer.

Supplements

I'm fortunate to have found a top immunologist who has had years of outstanding success with prostate cancer patients. Jesse uses powerful immune stimulants only after he had "fed" the immune system and improved the antioxidant status of the body first.

These supplements are absolutely vital to my total well being. Here's my daily regimen. It may look daunting, but remember: this is a war, and I'll do whatever it takes to win it.

1. PC SPES—An eight herb Chinese formulation which is critically important in reducing PSA scores.
2. A unique, comprehensive "food state" multi-vitamin and mineral formula that contains only 100% pure food. The most recent research shows that no nutrient can be delivered to your body's cells without the benefit of the naturally occurring co-factors found in food. Regular vitamins do not contain these vital food factors.
3. Antigen-infused dialyzable bovine colostrum whey extract. This immune system modulator has been prescribed by Dr. Stoff for all his patients who have a weakened immune system.
4. Plant sterols and sterolins are found abundantly in all fruits, vegetables, nuts, and seeds. These powerful substances have been developed by Professor Bouic as an effective agent to repair and normalize immune function in an easy-to-take capsule.
5. Cernitin flower pollen extract. This formula has been used extensively in Europe and Japan for prostate problems.
6. Coenzyme Q-10—A very potent antioxidant compound effective for heart disease and as an immune system enhancer. It is now used extensively for cancer. Coenzyme Q-10 levels decline in our bodies as we age and using it appears to increase energy levels in older people. Cancer patients appear to have low levels of Coenzyme Q-10.
7. Selenium has been clinically tested and proven to be effective in both preventing and stopping prostate cancer growth. This mineral is an absolute must in cancer protocol.

8. Lycopene is the unique substance found in tomatoes and tomato-based sauces, which have proved effective against prostate cancer.

9. Shark liver oil, taken from sharks caught in deep, cold waters, contains generous amounts of alkgycerol and squalene. These hard to get substances are also in human mothers' milk and help the newborn to have an effective and powerful immune system.

10. Natural Killer Cell Support Complex is available in a powdered form. This provides essential biochemical support for normal functioning of killer cells.

11. A liquid tonic for the immune system, which contains important special herbs, botanicals, and potassium.

12. Vitamin D 3. Many studies now show that men who have low levels of this vitamin have increased risk for prostate cancer. I alternate using an emulsified and gel form. I take 400 IUs daily.

13. Vitamin E is the principal fat soluble antioxidant protecting the body's cells. I take 800 IUs every day.

14. Additionally, because gluthione is so necessary for health, I take three supplements which help the body manufacture and utilize gluthione—they are cysteine, alpha-lipoic and n-acetyl cysteine. It has been noted by many physicians that if you have low levels of gluthione, you will almost certainly be sick. Conversely, high levels indicate wellness. I also recently discovered a superb supplement containing beet root, black currant, European elderberry, bilberry, and L-cysteine, which collectively raises gluthione levels.

15. Rhodiola rosea is an adaptogen more powerful than ginseng. It helps to normalize prostate fluids. This product when combined with another adaptogen, schisandra chinesis, helps to remove toxins from the liver.

16. Enzymes. Studies increasingly demonstrate their necessary involvement in total body health and anti-cancer activity.

17. Grape seed or pine bark. These polyphenolic compounds are the most powerful protective agents which are found in red wine.

18. Beta 1,3 glucan. Studies in Japan and the U.S. show this has strong anti-cancer action.

19. Maitake mushroom extract. I take 6–12 drops daily of this standardized form of beta-glucan. Again, many studies show this to be an effective agent against cancer.
20. Ipriflavone. This supplement, when combined with calcium, appears to increase bone density. Men who suffer from metastatic prostate cancer (as I do) will often experience loss of bone density.
21. Astragalus. This Chinese herb functions as an immune system enhancer.
22. Vitamin C. I use 2–4 grams daily. There is no doubt this vitamin is just as important today for immune health as it was for "Limeys" serving in England's navy in the 17th century. Vitamin C also protects DNA and cell proteins and membranes from free radicals.
23. A sublingual Vitamin B formulation, which revitalizes my energy levels in midafternoon just when I begin to falter. Vitamin B complex enormously helps in repair of DNA, the breakdown of which is strongly associated with cancer.
24. Modified citrus pectin. In studies, this powdered supplement may help prevent the spread of prostate cancer.

The above listing may seem to be overly extensive and expensive, as well. Well, yes, I take quite a few supplements and they are expensive. But, considering I take no hormones or drugs and have not had radiation or chemotherapy, I strongly believe the above-listed supplements have contributed enormously to my current well being and apparent control of my cancer.

Please refer to the resource section for additional information on this listing and where to obtain these supplements.

Avoiding Toxins

Obviously, we are all exposed to an overwhelming amount of toxins over which we have little or no control. There are approximately 100,000 synthetic chemicals in use today. We are faced with the awesome reality, for example, that 80 percent of pesticides have *not* been tested for safety!

Unfortunately we all have toxic chemicals deposited within our fatty tissues. But we can significantly slow down the amount of chemicals going into our bodies. With a bit of knowledge and steely determination, we can eliminate or reduce many chemicals from our lives. As a cancer victim, I have become viligant to possible sources of poisons in my life and will avoid these at all costs! Here's what you can do to minimize toxins in your system.

1. Purchase and use only organic fruits, vegetables, grains, etc. Do not be discouraged if your local greengrocer does not sell organic. If you look, you will find many sources. Buying organic is like buying a health insurance policy, one that pays off in staying healthy instead of getting sick.

2. Use only free range chickens and poultry. They're usually raised on antibiotic and hormone-free feed. Many health food stores now carry natural meat and fowl. If you can't find it locally, there are listings in the resource section of this book for some excellent mail order houses.

3. Use shampoos, soaps, shaving creams, toothpastes, after shave lotions, etc., that are as chemical free as possible. These are also available in your health food store.

4. Eliminate or reduce plastics that can come in contact with your food. Especially avoid cling wrap plastics, which can contain carcinogens.

5. Indulge in a purified water home filter system that can pull out most of the contaminants and such things as heavy metal that may be present in your municipal water supply system, or consider bottled water sources that have been purified and enhanced with bioavailable minerals and electrolytes.

6. Install a chlorine filter onto your shower head. Chlorine is not only absorbed through the skin, but vaporizes in the shower, and is inhaled directly into your lungs.

7. Replace all your powerful household cleaners that contain potentially carcinogenic chemicals. This includes your laundry and dishwasher detergents. Once again, your health food store usually carries safe and effective replacements.

8. Store no insecticides or pesticides in your residence, and do not allow any to be sprayed on your property.

9. If you have a choice, use wooden floors instead of carpets in

your home. The outgassing of chemicals from carpets is continual.

10. Do not jog or walk along heavily used automotive roadways. You don't need to breathe in noxious fumes.

11. Avoid microwaved and fried foods.

12. Keep your teeth and gums infection free. Infections from your mouth absolutely affect other areas of your body. Toxins are dangerous whether they come from outside or within your body.

13. Avoid and replace mercury fillings. Sweden and other European countries have observed the danger from mercury fillings and have begun to ban their use.

14. I've replaced all my beddings, which are synthetic or have feathers or plastics. My sheets, pillow cases, indeed even my pillow fillings, are all cotton.

15. Use household air filters and plants that actually filter your air supply.

16. Keep yourself happy and busy and avoid "toxic" negative or depressing thoughts.

Were most things better before prostate cancer? Without a doubt, physically, yes they were. But I have to be honest. In large part because my cancer has made me look up from the blur of responsibilities which had been my life, my relationship with my wife and children has become much richer. My wife, Roberta, became a strong partner in my healing, and her constant support helped clear the way to a faster recovery. She never stopped being a loving wife, despite my faltering libido.

Now, I have learned to enjoy aspects of my existence I never even noticed before. Now, I take walks, enjoy the sunshine whenever I have the chance, watch comedies, and try new things. And I have a new appreciation of my wonderful wife and partner, who supported me in every way.

Life is good, and Jesse has played a large role in keeping it that way. It is Jesse's conviction that the body can heal if we just give it a little help and allow it to do so. Improving the quality of life is an important part of that healing process.

Thank you, Jesse.

Afterword

It is now early March of the new millennium. Just nearly one year ago, I was diagnosed with prostate cancer, which had metastasized. At that time my Gleason score was a virulent 8. In the past twelve months, I learned to change many things in my life: the food I eat, the supplements I take, the toxins I avoid. Above all, I learned to adopt new, healthier and happier attitudes.

And now, I hold in my hand the latest report from Sloan Kettering, showing "no measurable amounts" of cancer in my PSA reading. The doctors call this score of 0.03 "undetectable." Remember, I had a rising PSA of 39.1 in April 1999. Additionally, a new CAT scan and bone scan indicate that my metastases have not spread and my lymph nodes are clear. All this without the use of any drug, chemotherapy or radiation.

In my war against prostate cancer, the battles have so far gone my way, but the war is still not over. Today, I feel physically terrific and emotionally unafraid and whatever happens, I will appreciate each day as a very precious gift.

PART TWO

A Return
to Balance

CHAPTER SIX

Restoring Immune Power

We cannot understand the body completely without taking history and culture into account. . . . The lonely individual suffering from the uncanny power of some strange ailment should realize that he is troubled in part by the unlived life of a collective which has dreamed his body process into being.

—Arnold Mindell

Case Study: Bill C. is a 62-year-old retired minister who was recovering from ankylosing spondylitis when he was found to have an early prostate cancer. Since alternative therapies were already helping him, he chose to start with other such therapies for his prostate cancer. He began with PC SPES, food state multivitamin, shark liver oil, flower pollen extracts, CO Q10, selenium, plant sterols and sterolins, AIDBCWE, acupuncture, and massage therapy. Over the next three months, his PSA dropped from 16.8 to 0.4. Now over a year in remission, his blood chemistry profiles and bone scan remain within normal ranges. He has decided to forgo retirement, and has once again become very active in his community, running support groups for people suffering from severe and chronic diseases, and helping to "break in" new ministers in surrounding churches.

Commentary: Much of what I do is remedial in that I prescribe substances to help normalize the immune function by supplying essential nutrients. As in the case of Bill C., such simple procedures, along with PC SPES, may be enough to place the cancer in remission. I often find myself counseling patients along the following lines: "Your immune system, had it been working normally, would have protected you. There are five reasons your immune system might have failed to protect you. First is direct trauma to your immune system, as would happen if you were exposed to radiation. Second is stress, and we'll talk more about that later. Third is infection, as by a virus that can attack and damage your immune system before it has a chance to fight back. We'll come back to this later, too. Fourth reason is a possible nutritional deficiency that would lead to an underpowered immune system. Fifth might be a toxin that's poisoning your system.

Your immune system is composed of many different types of cells, some of which divide rapidly when stimulated, thus consuming many nutrients in a short period of time.

The four issues we have to look at are: (1) an actual dietary deficiency that may have led to a deficiency in your body's store of immune "building blocks," (2) a relative deficiency due to a damaged digestive tract (very common as we age) preventing you from absorbing nutrients from your foods and supplements, (3) a secondary enzyme deficiency preventing you from using the nutrients in your foods, (4) a toxin that is interfering with your nutrients' actions directly, or which prevents an enzyme that is supposed to work with them from doing its job. In any case, if your system is suffering from a deficiency, it simply can't work right.

Correcting Nutritional Deficiencies

Under "normal" circumstances, when you're healthy and not under physical or mental stress, your system's requirements for nutrients can probably be met by a well-balanced organic food diet.

Now, let's get back to reality. Given the *toxins* in our air, food, and water supply, all of which require extra nutrients for the body to detoxify and eliminate them, and our usual, fast-paced, *stressed-out,*

Western lifestyle which also burns extra nutrients, even if we are eating whole, organic foods, virtually *all* of us wind up with a long list of nutritional deficiencies. Thus, the need for appropriate, focused supplementation to help maintain the normal foundation of our biochemistry so that it, in turn, can support our guardian immune system.

Research in this field is no longer confined to the practitioners of alternative and complementary medicine, but is now an area of intense interest in many conventional circles. For example, in the recent textbook, *Molecular Biology of Prostate Cancer,* the authors state,

> A new concept of dietary prevention of carcinoma of the prostate is based on epidemiological, biochemical, as well as on molecular biological studies. The degradation products from isoflavonoid-containing soy and high lignan-containing flax seed oil, which are also called phytochemicals, act as weak estrogens and seem to compete with testosterone and endogenous estrogens. Apart from being antiestrogenic—since they may also restrain the development of female breast cancer—they have also been called "natural tamoxifen."

Flaxseed *(Linum usitatissimum)*, for example, is a great source of dietary lignans. Lignans are a group of sugar-like molecules that combine with cellulose to form the cell wall of plants. They are found primarily in the woody tissues (like the seeds) of plants. Since the lignans are antiestrogenic, they compete with the natural estrogens our bodies make and, perhaps more importantly, with the xenoestrogens (not true estrogens, but estrogen-acting molecules which usually have health-damaging effects) that infiltrate our environment from pesticides, solvents, adhesives, soap emulsifiers, PCBs, etc. In order for the lignans to work in this beneficial way, they must be metabolized by the normal microflora in our digestive tracts.

The lignans found in flaxseed oil form fibrous chains that hold toxins in the intestinal tract and colon. Research has shown that patients with prostate and other cancers demonstrate a dramatic lowering of lignan content in bodily wastes when compared to noncancerous individuals. This suggests that phenolic lignan compounds help boost the immune response and detoxification of many metabolic processes. Animal studies show that flaxseed has directly demon-strated several anticarcinogenic effects.

Another antitumor effect comes from the omega-3 essential fatty acids (EFAs) that flaxseed oil contains. The two major members of the long-chain omega-3 group are EPA (eicosapentaenoic acid) and DHA (docosahexaenoic acid). Both are found in oil-rich fish like sardine, mackerel, pilchard, herring, and salmon and in cod liver oil. (The cod itself is not a good source of omega-3s, yet its liver pro-vides excellent supplies of both EPA and DHA.) EPA is manufac-tured in our body from alpha-linolenic acid—the primary fatty acid in flaxseed oil—when everything is working the way it is supposed to. Unfortunately, it doesn't work well enough when someone has cancer. Thus, it is a good idea to supplement with some fish oils even when supplementing with flaxseed oil. These oils are somewhat fragile, so once opened, bottles should be kept out of the sunlight and in the refrigerator.

Overconsumption of "bad" highly saturated fats and trans-fats (such as are found in fried foods), and diets that are low in essential fatty acids (EFAs), result in fat deposits leading to obesity and fatty degeneration. When "good" unsaturated fats rich in EFAs enhance energy production, less fat is deposited. The richest source of omega-3 fatty acids is flaxseed oil, with 55–65 percent omega-3 and 15–25 per-cent omega-6 fatty acids. However, about 80 percent of the American population is believed to be deficient in omega-3 fatty acids.

EFAs and their derivatives serve a number of vital functions, in-cluding the transport and metabolism of cholesterol and triglycerides, support of normal brain development and function (from the phos-pholipids it contains), and maintenance of the structure of cell mem-branes (antiwrinkle effect). EFAs increase the metabolic rate, oxygen uptake, and energy production; slow down the growth of cancer cells, enhance immune function, and increase the production of "good" prostaglandins to help prevent blood clots and reduce inflammation.

Enhancing Enzyme Strength

Essential fatty acids and other important nutrients don't work all by themselves—they are carefully inserted in place with the help of enzymes, special proteins that occur in all living things and are essential for life. Medical researchers have identified more than 2,700 different enzymes in the body, which help our bodies repair damage, generate immune responses, grow, break down and digest our food, and fight cancer.

Enzymes working in tandem operate like a construction crew on a conveyer belt: A becomes B, which is converted to C and D, etc. Generally speaking, the sum total of these enzymatic reactions is our metabolism. Our bodies contain millions of enzymes, which continually repair, maintain and protect us. Many people have never heard about enzymes and are unaware of their importance in regulating their bodies and maintaining their health.

Each of these activities requires energy, which becomes available from the activity of our enzymes. Without energy, cells become disorganized, resulting in an increased risk of cancer, other illnesses, and even death.

This observation was carefully studied and reported upon by Dr. Otto Warburg in 1926, and we're still trying to figure out how to best make use of this information. Normal cells utilize oxygen as part of the biochemical reactions that take apart sugar and other nutrients to produce energy, and lots of it. As a byproduct of this energy production, heat is released, thus our body's temperature of 98.6 +/− 1 degrees. Within our cells, energy is produced and used mainly in the form of adenosine triphosphate (ATP). ATP is used throughout the cell to energize (like the bunny) or power virtually all of the intracellular metabolic reactions, including those of cell division. Normal cell division uses up a lot of energy and depends on the normal function of a number of important enzymes, some of which are dependant on hormones, like the thyroid hormones, messenger proteins, like calmodulin (which is produced inside most of our cells), and minerals, like calcium. This leads to the topic of vitamin D and its role in getting calcium into the cells where it is needed and calmodulin inhibiters as potential anti-cancer agents, which I will touch on in my discussion of vitamin D.

Cancer cells don't rely upon the availability of oxygen to help fuel their metabolic reactions. They use sugar as a fuel source and disassemble it into lactic acid, not carbon dioxide and water, like normal cells do. This is why sugar must be avoided in your diet!

Energy manufactured by cancer cells is considerably lower than that produced in normal tissues, which is why ancient Chinese physician/herbalists referred to cancer as a "cold" disease.

Anticancer diets eliminate sugar and refined carbohydrates, in part because when you eat foods rich in these items, it creates a fuel source readily available to cancer cells. Lactic acid builds up in the tissues around the cancer, and is a chief cause of the pain associated with cancer. As lactic acid builds up, it makes the tissues more acidic, which leads to enzyme dysfunction. The problem becomes, "How can we *selectively* block the abnormal, defective, and inefficient metabolism of cancer cells without affecting normal cell metabolism?"

One way is to stop supporting the existence of the cancer cells, or to selectively starve them out! At the same time, the operative word is *selectively*, so that a particular inhibitor does not disrupt vital, normal body processes such as the beating of our hearts or the process of breathing. (We need to be careful to not create a dreaded "side effect.")

Such strategies are considered when working on "antimetabolite" chemotherapeutic drugs. Some plants produce substances that have antimetabolite effects. These often are highly purified into drugs (with attendant side effects), such as Taxol.

Enzymes play several other important roles in the fight against cancer. If your immune system is functioning normally and can "see" a cancer cell, it will destroy it. Part of the problem which leads to the accumulation of cancer cells into a tumor is that these cancer cells are able to "cloak" themselves from the vigilantes of the immune system. This cloaking device is based on the varied surface structures of the tumor cells. They are not recognized as being "nonself," and thus vulnerable to attack by the immune system warriors. Cancers also release blocking proteins into the bloodstream as a smoke screen to blind the immune system. Furthermore, invasive cancer processes and the formation of metastases are, to an extent, dependent on the stickiness of the blood. People with cancer are more likely to develop blood clots, hence, again the recommendation for essential fatty acids. Adding fuel to the fire, the cancer cells themselves are "stickier" than normal cells.

Research has shown that tumor cells also use fibrin, or clotting proteins, to camouflage their typical cell-surface landmarks to avoid recognition as foreign by the immune system. Removing or breaking down the fibrin decreases the development of metastases and makes the cancer cells more vulnerable to attack by the immune system.

By taking enzymes that digest fibrin (best between meals), it is possible to reduce the stickiness of the cancer cells and to decrease their invasive and unruly behavior. Some enzyme preparations available today have a good track record when it comes to helping in the fight against cancer because they are active both in the gastrointestinal tract and in the blood.

Their success may be linked to taking specially coated enzymes derived from natural plant sources. These contain:

- *Lipase* for digesting fats.
- *Amylase* for digesting starches.
- *Protease* for digesting protein.
- *Cellulase* for the digestion of plant cellulose.
- *Lactase* for digesting dairy products.

The study of the importance of enzymes and of their flip side, heartburn, has become a worldwide concern. According to Dr. James B. Summer, Nobel Prize Winner and Professor of Biochemistry, Cornell University, and the author of "The Secrets of Life Enzymes," $5 billion a year is being spent on blocking acid production even though our ability to produce acid usually peaks around age eleven! So why do we remove stomach acid with antacids or repress it by using acid blockers? We are treating symptoms! One perceived symptom, "excess stomach acid," is caused by stomach acid splashing up into the esophagus, which is protected by the lower esophageal sphincter (LES). The esophagus does not have the alkaline mucous that your stomach has to protect its walls. So when the LES does not work adequately, acid splashing up gives the burning sensation of "heartburn."

Taking antacids and acid blockers alters the body's natural processes. Stomach acid is important for digesting food (its production tends to decrease as we age). It activates digestive enzymes and discourages many detrimental microbes. When you remove stomach acid with antacids or prevent its production with acid blockers, you are altering natural digestion and making it difficult to get the nutrients from your food and supplements.

Effective digestion requires enzymes to absorb the nutrients in food and supplements. Enzymes are an important part of the therapeutic strategy!

Enzyme quantities and activity in your gastrointestinal tract can decrease for many different reasons, including aging, nutritional deficiencies, local damage, infection or inflammation of the gastrointestinal tract. Many factors influence the overgrowth of harmful bacteria and can cause an infection in the gastrointestinal tract. Studies have shown that people whose diets contain high amounts of animal products and little vegetable fiber are more likely to develop gastrointestinal diseases. Refined sugar, refined white flour, and other highly refined carbohydrates can also disrupt the gastrointestinal tract and lead to a bacterial imbalance. Taking antibiotics, which often kill good bacteria along with the bad bacteria, is another cause of bacterial imbalance in the gastrointestinal tract. Antibiotics can be life-saving, but should used only when necessary.

Antibiotics: Pro and Con

In 1928, Sir Alexander Fleming discovered a revolutionary way of successfully dealing with sicknesses caused by infections of unfriendly bacteria. That landmark discovery was penicillin, the first antibiotic to be prescribed for life-threatening bacterial infections. Most doctors at the time were quite convinced that penicillin and similar antibiotics would prove to be the panacea (magic bullet) for all infections and ultimately lead to the end of all infectious diseases. Unfortunately, infectious diseases haven't been eradicated, despite the specialized antibiotics on the market today. The fact is, no matter how strong or continuously antibiotics are applied, they simply can't kill off every single bad bacterium, and those that survive will be resistant to the antibiotics used.

Antibiotics, when properly prescribed, are important medical tools that save many lives. But antibiotics are among the most overly and inappropriately prescribed drugs. For example, antibiotics are useless against the common cold and other virus illnesses, which are not affected by antibiotic treatment. Many common ailments such as fevers, earaches, and sore throats are called "self-limiting." This means, when they occur in most healthy people, the immune system should be able to easily overcome the ailment. In the process of beating the ailment, the immune system should emerge stronger and theoretically able to resist or beat that ailment again. The use of antibiotics in cases of self-limiting infections, especially for viral infections, is usually inappropriate. Worse even than the inappropriate use of antibiotics in humans is the extremely widespread use of antibiotics in livestock and poultry. Bacteria that develop a resistance to antibiotics can sometimes pass on that resistance to other types of bacteria, which argues for radically restricting the use of antibiotics to medically valid cases.

We can help our own immune systems by increasing the number of friendly *Bifidobacteria* and *Lactobacilli* in our lower gastrointestinal tracts. This can be done with supplements. These and other important microorganisms are the keys to putting our whole system in order and restoring the vital ability of the gastrointestinal tract to absorb the nutrients that we need.

Over 75 percent of my prostate cancer patients report gastrointestinal problems to me, including gas, bloating, diarrhea, constipation, and abdominal cramping. Evaluating these problems with tests like a Comprehensive Digestive Stool Analysis, G.I. Evaluation Panel, colonoscopy, or other tests is vital in the face of such chronic complaints, lest the supplements later prescribed simply go in one end and out the other. Wherever there are G-I tract complaints, some degree of malabsorption exists which can lead to or intensify other problems, such as anemia.

Dietary Dos and Don'ts

While we're talking about the gastrointestinal tract, let's talk about one of my favorite subjects, food. What should cancer patients eat? What kind of diet is going to help? There are almost as many books on diets as there are tacos in Tucson. However, the best diet should have some very specific characteristics. It has to be high in quality nutrition, easy to digest, low in stressors to the liver to aid in detoxification, supportive to the immune system, reasonably easy to follow, and last, but not least, worth eating. Often I will recommend a specific diet for unusual circumstances, but usually I will start with a modified "Eat Right for Your Type" diet that works well for my patients.

Dr. Peter D'Adamo coauthored the bestselling book, *Eat Right for Your Type,* offering a diet strategy based upon your blood type. This book extends the research begun by his father, Dr. James D'Adamo, more than a dozen years ago. As it turns out, your blood type not only reflects many aspects of your internal biochemistry, but also influences protein and immunological interactions. Following a dietary strategy based upon your blood type will supply high-quality nutrition through a specific (and appetizing) selection of foods that will minimize stress on your immune system. Furthermore, by avoiding some of the foods that have a high fat content, you will minimize stress on your liver as well.

The scientific basis of this is established in the study of special proteins called lectins that are found in foods. An example of a lectin that has been used in the pursuit of medical science is a protein found in wheat called phytohemagglutinin (PHA). PHA is so named because it is a plant (phyto) protein that agglutinates (causes the clotting of) blood (heme). This is a general characteristic of lectins and the basis of the diet; avoid that which makes your blood thicker! Remember that thickness, stickiness and clots all tend to support metastatic activity. Some lectins also stimulate cell division, another good reason to avoid them. Lectins are a convenient way, owing to their stickiness, for micro-organisms to attach themselves to other organisms. Thus germs, and even some cells in our immune system, use this super-glue to their benefit. Special cells in our liver's bile ducts have lectins on their surface to help them snare roaming bacteria. When you eat a food that contains lectins that are incompatible with the protein lectins that your cells make for themselves, the lectins from the food will begin to agglutinate blood cells in and around various key organs such as your liver. Centuries ago when the ancient wise Chinese physician/herbalists spoke about stagnant liver chi, they were probably describing this kind of congesting process. They also described cancer not only as a "cold" disease, but as a "stagnant" one, as well.

Meanwhile, medical science marches forward. On a street corner in downtown London back in 1978, a KGB agent assassinated Gyorgi Markov while he waited for a bus. He wasn't shot, strangled, hung or clubbed but quietly stabbed by an object—perhaps an umbrella point—that inserted a tiny gold bead into his leg. The bead was permeated with a chemical called *ricin,* a highly poisonous substance extracted from caster beans. It is so potent that even an infinitesimally small dose can cause death, almost instantly, by rapidly converting circulating red blood cells into blood vessel-blocking clots. The moral to the story is this: to minimize the lectins in your diet that are stressful to your immune system, know your blood type—and avoid umbrella points!

Once you know your blood type, you have two priorities when choosing what to eat: (1) choose foods that are high in nutrient value to supply the basic building blocks your body needs to repair itself, and (2) choose foods that will relieve any additional stress on your liver and immune system. Your basic diet should be mostly vegetables, some whole grains, and some protein as per the blood type diet. If you really love ice cream and hot dogs, shift to moderate consumption.

On the list to "restrict or cut out completely" are red and most other meats—meaning beef, veal, lamb, and pork (some organically raised beef is occasionally OK for Type Os), all deep-fried foods, caffeine (coffee, tea except for special extracts, most soft drinks, chocolate), and alcohol. (A note on moderation: If you get drunk more than once a month, you are crossing the line from moderation into serious trouble no matter what your physical condition; if you're a weekend warrior, you're already in trouble.)

Dairy products should be limited to no more than a half glass of low-fat milk or a piece of cheese once every other week. Sugar should be avoided, or at most, limited to a couple of teaspoons per day. All of these substances either put a toxic stress on the body or slow down the immune system. Smoking, of course, is out.

Since most of us can't judge for ourselves what moderation is, especially after we have exceeded it, we will give you numbers to go by. You may treat yourself to one of the above restricted items (*not one of each!*) once every other week, or once every month if you can hold out that long. If you absolutely have to, you can allow yourself that special treat once a week. But don't exceed this limit. This is an important thing to remember, especially during the early stages of your retaliation against prostate cancer.

Remember, your diet and its absorption are *critical* to your recovery. Most of us eat a SAD diet that doesn't provide what's needed to fight the good fight. You never heard of SAD? Well, the SAD diet is the Standard American Diet, and given the epidemic of cancer and other severe and chronic diseases we're facing today, it's woefully inadequate. Not only is it high in toxins, it's low in vital nutrients, including minerals. For many decades it has been clear that minerals are critical to support our health and restore our immune system. Potassium, in particular, plays a prominent role in the counterattack against cancer. Dr. Max Gerson discovered this years ago and it has since proven its worth, especially regarding its relationship to salt.

Going back to our days in caves, we humans initially had to adapt to retain sodium from a sodium-poor diet and to excrete potassium from a potassium-rich, hunter-gatherer diet. We obviously have not yet reconciled our biology to today's high-sodium, low-potassium (SAD, junk) foods. The influence of the sodium-potassium ratio on cancer development—first discovered by epidemiological research—has been confirmed by various means, including:

- Dietary and biochemical studies (you are what you eat)
- Gerontological and biochemical studies (the effects of aging)
- Biochemical and cellular studies of relationships between hyper- and hypokalemic states and cancer (that is, too much and too little potassium)
- Reviews of cellular changes in relationship to this sodium/ potassium ratio as induced by carcinogenic agents
- Reviews of cellular changes in relationship to this ratio, as induced by anticarcinogenic agents
- Numerous animal experiments

Research shows that the high-sodium, low-potassium ratio increases in test animals with tumors. Other studies demonstrate that the shift in sodium and potassium across the cell membrane may play an integral role in the promotion of cancer. Over the years many different forms of potassium have been used to aid in the battle against cancer.

Here are some high-potassium foods to boost those levels:

- bananas
- dates
- papaya
- spinach
- garlic
- cantaloupe

One particular supplement I have found useful over the years due to its unique formulation is a blend of potassium, and other minerals, and extracts of healthful plants, flowers, foliage, roots, and barks. It contains five different forms of potassium, which together deliver 562 milligrams per 2 tablespoons (one dose) and is thus to be highly recommended. Over its 70-year history, studies of this supplement have shown it to be extremely immune-supportive. The herbal polysaccharides that it contains aid the functioning of the bone marrow and the immune system.

(For more information, see the Resource Section.)

When patients go on antiandrogen drugs, nutritional deficiencies and toxic side effects weaken bone marrow function in the later stages of prostate cancer, causing anemia, a decrease in your level of red blood cells. This in turn leads to fatigue, muscle weakness, shortness of breath, and a decreased ability of the blood to carry oxygen. Since cancer thrives in an oxygen-lacking environment, anemia will work against you on several fronts.

The use of iron supplements, in cases of severe anemia, must be handled very carefully. In the early stages of prostate cancer, most men seem to need some iron, since the immune system seems to burn it while fighting the cancer.

In the later stages of the disease, probably due to multiple organ dysfunctions, iron frequently becomes a burden to the body as it can wind up being stored and deposited as ferritin, a by-product that further stresses the body. Then, you'll need the B vitamins, which are critical to use up iron and produce blood. Much of iron's absorption depends on the normal functioning of our digestive tract and its micro-organisms. Thus, again, we must pay careful attention to our digestive processes and support them with extra acidophilus supplements and B complex. B vitamins are a usual constituent of a good multivitamin supplement. In addition to the B vitamins, the herb *Pulsatilla* is extremely useful in helping with anemia, fatigue, and the emotional vulnerability that often accompany that tired rotten anemic feeling. Your loved ones will appreciate your adding it to your regimen.

Certain oils can help protect and support your bone marrow and the production of red blood cells. In this case it's not snake oil, but shark liver oil that has proven to be helpful. The healing effects of shark oil on the tissues of the body have been confirmed in modern times through many clinical trials, most of which have been conducted by Swedish physicians and scientists. The biological effects of this oil are attributed to its content of certain substances, called *alkylglycerols*. These substances occur naturally in small amounts, primarily in our bone marrow, the liver, the spleen, and in mothers' milk (ten times more in human milk than in cow's milk). Shark liver oil comes from cold-water sharks and is particularly rich in alkyl-glycerols. The oil in this product has been standardized and extensively purified in order to qualify it for medical use and study. In the purification process, PCBs, pesticides, and heavy metals have been removed. The effects of alkylglycerols on the immune system and on cancer have been confirmed over the last 40 years through extensive research and clinical studies. I find them very helpful to stabilize anemia and protect the bone marrow in general.

The downward spiral of failing health, heralded by anemia, will, if unchecked, lead to the more severe condition of "cachexia," an advanced state of malnutrition that results in lean tissue wasting and marked weight loss. When left unchecked, it will kill much faster than cancer. It is directly responsible for somewhere between 22 to 67 percent of all cancer deaths! Laboratory testing shows up to 80 percent of all men with advanced prostate cancer have reduced levels of serum albumin, a leading indicator of protein and calorie malnutrition. Unbalanced dietary protein restriction (an unbalanced vegan diet) in someone with cancer does not affect the composition or growth rate or the tumors. It does reduce the quality and quantity of life of the patient, so watch your blood type and diet! This is why

I have a naturopathic physician on my staff and work with a clinical biochemist to help avoid such nutritional disasters. Cachexia occurs for many reasons, such as damage to the digestive tract, depression, malnutrition, and the added stress from the release of cytokines, which the immune system releases as it fights the cancer, specifically TNF-alpha.

There are other ways to knock out cachexia. One of the best ways is with aggressive nutritional support, including fish oils (EPA). One very important study showed that adding fish oils to the supplement regimen for cancer patients was extremely beneficial.

Another supplement (available by prescription only) found to be helpful against cachexia is hydrazine sulfate. Human clinical studies at the University of California at Los Angeles showed it reduced lean body weight loss and improved the abnormal glucose and insulin levels common in late-stage cancer patients. A more elegant way of not only reversing cachexia and rearming the immune system is to give intravenous TNF-beta, which will block abnormal TNF-alpha production. Tumor Necrosis Factor-beta (trade name Kinetrex™) has been in clinical use and trials since the mid 1970s by one of the founding fathers of clinical immunology, Dr. Ben Papermaster. It has proven to be an invaluable aid to many patients who either have a dysfunctional "sleeping" immune system, cachexia, or both. Since much of the bone pain associated with this advanced metastatic cancer is eased by TNF-alpha, giving TNF-beta will help that, too, and without any toxic side effects!

Surviving in a Toxic World

Speaking of toxic side effects, what exactly is a toxin? A toxin is any substance that, when present in the body in a sufficient quantity, damages an organ, system, or function. A toxin is usually thought of as something that comes from outside of us. But this is not true. Someone with liver or kidney failure can die from the adverse effects of the toxins that accumulate from their own biochemical processes. To a lesser extent, if these organs aren't working optimally, the person can still become sluggish and/or sick. Most toxins adversely affect one or more enzyme functions, but the most serious effects are those that in some way affect our DNA and the process of cell division, which can actually cause cancer.

It is difficult to avoid toxins because they are found everywhere. The noted authority Samuel Epstein, M.D., of the University of Illinois says that a major thrust of cancer prevention must be the detoxification of our earth. (We'll come to detoxifying ourselves in a moment.) Toxins not only cause DNA breakage, which can trigger cancer, but also weaken and compromise immune function, which then allows cancer to become the "fox in the chicken coop" with no controlling force. Early research indicated that once cancer has been up-regulated, or the lion is "out of the cage," then no amount of detoxification (by itself) is going to matter.

Through his intensive research, Dr. Bruce Ames of the University of California at Berkeley, California, has estimated that each of the 60 trillion cells in our body undergoes from 1,000 to 10,000 DNA "hits" or potentially cancer-causing breaks every day! For most of us, our DNA enzyme repair mechanisms and immune system surveillance by our natural killer cells are able to keep this storm of potentially deadly genetic damage under control.

Dr. Patrick Quillin, Vice-President of Cancer Treatment Centers of America, has written about many of the sources of these carcinogenic toxins and lists them as coming from these sources:

TOXINS, TOXINS EVERYWHERE

Voluntary pollutants:

Drugs. Drug abuse is an absolute epidemic, especially in our inner cities. Not only can the abuse lead to damage in the immune system, and other organs depending upon the type of drug and method of administration, but drug overdose and the trauma related to drug trafficking activities is the number one cause of death in the 14–21-year-old population in most cities in the United States.

Alcohol. In addition to being a direct toxin to the digestive tract, liver, brain, kidneys and pancreas, alcohol is also a very powerful solvent. As such it can bring many other allergens, toxins, and chemicals directly into the body that wouldn't have otherwise been absorbed if they weren't mixed in with a "drink or two." This can lead to a broad spectrum of diseases ranging from mixed chemical sensitivity to cancer, depending upon what other toxins it is potentiating. It's best left as a cleaning fluid and not as a source of liquid refreshment.

Tobacco. What can we say—have you read the newspapers lately? Tobacco products, in addition to being a delivery system for nicotine, a highly addictive drug, are carcinogenic. Diseases like emphysema, heart attacks, strokes, and peripheral vascular disease are "light-weights" compared to the misery of throat and mouth cancer, stomach cancer, and lung cancer. If you smoke, please see the light and don't reach for one.

Involuntary Toxins from:
Food. 1.2 billion pounds of pesticides are dumped on fresh produce; there are 2,800 FDA-approved food additives; and 5 million pounds of antibiotics are used each year to grow animals faster. In addition, our food contains herbicides, fungicides, wax on produce, parasites, veterinarian drug residue, and hormones.

Water. The EPA estimates that 40 percent of the fresh water in the United States is unusable; and 1,300 different chemicals exist in the average "EPA-approved" city drinking water. Chlorine and lead are most common, with many industrial volatile organic chemicals ending up in the drinking water. 60,000 chemicals are in regular use, according to the American Chemical Society, and half of these are in regular contact with humans, of which at least 20,000 are known carcinogens, or cancer-causing agents. Other toxins are found in the farm runoff of herbicides, pesticides, fertilizer (nitrates combine with amino acids in the stomach to form carcinogenic nitrosamines).

Air. Fifty million Americans breathe air that is dangerous for health. Smoking and secondhand smoke are obvious. Millions of tons of known carcinogens are produced annually and legally from paper mills, petrochemical refineries, burning of medical waste (generate dioxin from PVC), crop dusting, diesel fumes, leaded exhaust, etc.

Industrial exposure. Workers in factories are exposed to toxins in the vinyl industry, paper mills, refineries, asbestos, etc.

Household products. Cleaners, and the like. See *The Safe Shopper's Bible* by D. Steinman et.al.

Other. Mercury amalgams, electromagnetic fields from cellular phone antennas, high-voltage power lines.

Recent evidence shows that detoxification does work. Cancer growth can be slowed and even reversed under the right conditions of detoxification. According to the National Cancer Institute, there are 7 million Americans who are alive today 5 or more years after their cancer diagnosis.

If toxins cause cancer, then detoxification is an important part of the solution. The first step of detoxification is to avoid further toxin exposure.

However, this is easier said than done! Let's take water, for example. Half the toxins in water come from what they add to it to neutralize the other toxins already there, or to confer some ill-conceived health benefit. Fluoride is an extremely powerful enzyme inhibitor and a waste product of the aluminum and phosphate fertilizer industries. It's added to the water to give us stronger teeth and bones. Maybe if we all drank fewer soft drinks and ate less sugar, it wouldn't have been an issue to begin with, but be that as it may, fluoride is only a political answer. Currently, much to the chagrin of all of the authorities involved, in-depth testing of the Tucson water supply showed the presence of radon, a gas released from radioactive mineral deposits. Now, the powers-that-be are trying to figure what a "safe" level of radon is in a water supply! I'll just keep drinking my purified bottled water regardless of the final political answer.

> Everything causes cancer? Perhaps. Conceivably even a single electron at the other side of the universe. The real question is, how likely is any one particular cause? In point of fact, fluoride causes more human cancer death, and causes it faster, than any other chemical.
>
> —Dean Burk, Chief Chemist Emeritus
> U.S. National Cancer Institute

Our food isn't much better. Pesticides and antibiotics in our foods have estrogenic effects (are xenoestrogens) and are directly implicated in both breast and prostate cancer. Food additives such as BHA, BHT, Food Dye Red No. 3, Blue No. 2, Green No. 3, Citrus Red No. 2, propyl gallate, and sodium nitrite all fuel the cancer maelstrom. The depletion of the soil across our agricultural belt has left our food nutritionally hollow, a mere façade of its intended value. Since the advent of synthetic fertilizers, the protein content of our vegetable staples has dropped by 50 percent! Needless to say, I recommend only organic or biodynamically raised produce.

We can discuss for hours the toxins in our home sweet homes. Formaldehyde gas is high on the list as a common toxin in our homes as a result of outgassing from carpeting and many common building materials. Our castles have become our nemesis and not our protector from the harsh reality around us. You can run, but you can't hide.

After looking in horror at the toxic load forced upon us, the question is not, "Why do one-third of us get cancer?" but more appropriately, "Why do *only* one-third of us get cancer?" Regardless of other measures taken, our cancer epidemic will not abate until we get our environment cleaned up. Increasing our ability to purge poisons through detoxification may help some cancer patients recover. Vital to detoxification are antioxidants such as vitamin E and selenium. In fact, right down the road from my house, Dr. Larry C. Clark's group did a preventive study and reported that selenium treatment brought a 63 percent reduction in prostate cancer occurrence!!

However, all selenium is not created equally. The selenium that they and several other researchers used was a yeast-converted selenium that is extremely bioavailable, safe, and consistent.

The prostate gland seems to be very sensitive to the effects of selenium with the assistance of vitamin E. So, in addition to the positive effects that selenium has on prostate cancer, its detox effects are nothing short of miraculous. Again, this is critical because the toxic burden that we bear can cripple our immune systems, scramble our DNA, adversely alter our cellular functions, and promote cancer growth.

As an individual, there are things that you can do *today* to lighten the toxic millstone we all share. You can start drinking bottled water from a reputable, certified company, at least 8 eight-ounce glasses per day. You can also increase your fiber intake by adding psyllium seeds or, preferably, ground flaxseeds to your diet. Products such as modified citrus pectin will also help in absorb toxins from your digestive tract. If constipation is an issue, get it fixed *now.* Acupuncture, herbal laxatives, enemas, and colonics (occasionally) are all helpful, and while we're on the subject, let's talk about coffee enemas, the *only* approved use of coffee I recommend.

Coffee enemas help to purge the colon and liver of accumulated toxins and dead tissue. Coffee enemas are prepared by brewing regular organic and caffeinated coffee, let cool to body temperature, then use enema bag as per instructions with 4 to 8 ounces of the coffee solution. Proponents of this therapy use it daily for very sick cancer patients, or weekly for recovering cancer patients.

—Dr. Patrick Quillin, *Beating Cancer with Nutrition*

I have found coffee enemas to be *extremely helpful* in quickly relieving detox symptoms that may occur, for example, as a tumor starts to break up under the counterattack of the immune system. Given how odd this recommendation sounds to many people, I usually let one patient recommend it to another as they sit side by side getting various intravenous therapies. Then I merely have to confirm its truth and I don't get the strange looks anymore. At a slower pace, there is a wonderful herbal combination to gently help detoxify your system (see Resource Section). Talk to your physician about other areas that may need to be detoxified, such as heavy metals. One controversial area of toxicity is that of dental amalgam fillings and root canals. Space does not permit an in-depth discussion of all of the pros and cons on this subject, but suffice it to say that I wouldn't recommend getting any more of these fillings should you already have a collection.

Unbeknownst to most of us, our lives hang precariously close to disaster. Of course, those with cancer already know it. We have reached the point wherein we *must* clean up our act . . . or risk extinction. As master Yoda said, it is time to "Do or do not. There is no 'try.' "

CHAPTER SEVEN

Boosting the Immune System

Reduced natural killer cell activity is present in all illness.
—Dr. Lewis L. Lanier of DNAX Research, as quoted in *Immunity*

All cancers are associated with decreased immune function. The fact that some aspect of immune suppression can be found in most people in our society today does not make it normal nor does it bode well for the future of mankind.
—Dr. Yulius Poplyansky, Director of the International Foundation for Innovative Medicine

Case Study: Jurgen S. is a 65-year-old master goldsmith who was diagnosed with a prostate abnormality at his yearly physical. A biopsy showed it to be an early prostate cancer. His PSA on diagnosis was only 12.4 and he was otherwise symptom-free. Because he was familiar with integrative medicine, he chose to use alternative approaches first. I began with my standard protocol of supplements, along with supportive homeopathic remedies, natural killer cell complex, and grapeseed. Over the next three months, his PSA dropped to 0.9. It remained in that area over the next eight months while he gradually decreased and then stopped the injections. He remained on the supplements. Now, six years later, he does a round of injections 6 weeks in the spring and fall and continues to be in remission.

Commentary: The successful involvement of the immune system is fundamental to controlling cancers, and there are many different ways to accomplish this reactivation. We must first take a closer look at the frontline of the immune defense: the blood. In the time that you began reading this chapter, your body has created some 4 million new immune cells and hundreds of thousands of antibody molecules! Such massive production may seem overzealous until you consider that even if you are perfectly healthy, thousands of viruses may be present in your blood, only about 75 percent of which have been identified. Some of these viruses are implicated in prostate cancer.

How the Immune System Works

The immune system works by circulating "warriors," or cells, that are capable of acting far from their points of origin. The complexity of this system rivals that of the nervous system, and in fact the similarities between the two are quite real. It is no accident of nature that the thymus gland, the bone marrow, and the lymph nodes—all major centers of immunity—are bundled in ropes of nerves. The brain is known to transmit both electrical and chemical signals along nerves to stimulate and amplify immune responses. As the signals stream out from the brain, they often pass warnings from the immune centers flying in the opposite direction.

The immune system is not merely a tool manipulated by the brain; it is a sensory organ as well. It transmits chemical messages about bacteria, fungi, viruses, bits of dead tissue, and cancer cells. (Cancer cells, by the way, seem to arise every day in everybody and must be disposed of before they can accumulate to the point of becoming a tumor.) The wonder of it all is that such organization is possible, with the use of only a few distinct cell types whose members are widely scattered throughout the body.

Most immune cells originate in bone marrow, a soft, spongy material located at the centers of all major bones. Under a microscope, the most easily identifiable of all of the immune cells is the *macrophage*. Its nucleus (the part of the cell where DNA, the substance that directs all protein production, is contained) looks like a dark, horseshoe-shaped blob and occupies much of the space inside the cell. The macrophage is usually quite large compared to other cells of the immune system.

The Healing Scavengers

If you have ever played "Pac Man," the video arcade game, you will have a good idea of how the macrophage functions: it scavenges—chomp, chomp, chomp. The macrophages develop from stem cells in the bone marrow and in their infancy are called *monocytes*. Monocytes become macrophages when they are released into the blood and migrate into tissues. They then mature into large, amoeba-like eating machines. Local accumulations of macrophages in the body form a sort of network called the reticuloendothelial system (RES). Such accumulations are most prominent in the walls of the intestines, in the nervous system, spleen, lungs, and connective tissue. The greatest concentration of RES is in the liver, where the macrophages are known as *Kupffer cells* and play an active and important role in helping the liver with its detoxification duties. Indeed, Kupffer cells comprise about 10 percent of the liver's total mass. Macrophages also accumulate in tissues that are injured or inflamed, such as in arthritic joints. There they seek out infectious agents or irritants.

Like the amoeba, the macrophage pushes out lobes or tentacles, surrounds the offending cancer cell (or prey), and brings it into itself. Deep within the absorbed cell, enzymes are released. The prey is dismantled; its nutrients absorbed. After dining on a cancer cell, bacterium, or fungus, or on a large clump of viruses tied together by antibodies (the macrophage cannot "see" individual virus particles and handles only those packaged into large clumps by other cells), the macrophage "studies" it. Then it transmits chemical alarms that begin a whole cascade of immunological response, a call to arms!

One of the substances released is called *interleukin-6* (IL-6), a very powerful immune-activating biochemical produced and released by stimulated macrophages, as well as by the anterior lobe of the pituitary. The production of IL-6 can, however, be suppressed when someone is under an excessive level of stress for a prolonged period of time. Macrophages are said to "present" the toxin to the rest of the immune system to start the counterattack. B-cells then take up the message and direct antibody production against any interlopers that might still be wandering about. Natural killer cells and T-helper cells, too, are awakened to join the feast.

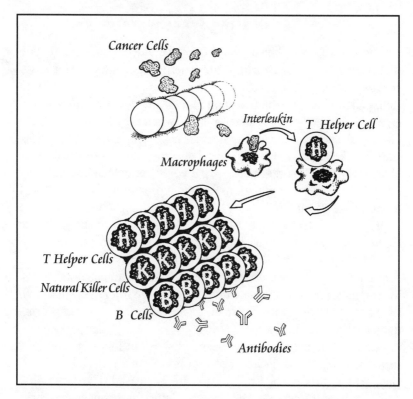

Figure 3. Marshalling the Troops. The body has powerful defenses. Most cancers never grow very large before they are attacked and destroyed by the immune system. One key to surviving an established cancer is to find ways of reactivating the body's immune responses.

Many different things can stimulate the activity of the macrophages. Two powerful stimulants that I use are BCG and glucan. The immune stimulant *Bacillus Calmette-Guerin* (BCG) helps break *anergy,* the nonreactivity of the immune system commonly found in patients with cancer. A second macrophage stimulant I use is Beta-1,3-polyglucose, otherwise known as Beta-1,3-D-Glucan. It is an extract from the cell wall of the yeast, *Saccharomyces cerevisae.* When given intralesionally or intravenously, it stimulates the bejesus out of the macrophages and starts the immune cascade off with a bang, thus fulfilling the first task of the immune system.

In order to function normally, the immune system must first *rec-*

ognize that something is amiss. Macrophages and their cousins, the dendritic cells, accomplish this recognition by releasing cytokines, or messenger molecules, thus sounding the alarm. The dendritic cells, thus named because of the long, thin, finger-like projections protruding from their surface, are the only nonmobile cells of the immune system. Newly discovered and largely mysterious, they sit, fixed in place, within our different tissues constantly "tasting" their environments for danger. When danger is sensed, for example, in the form of cellular damage, they "process and present" the offending antigen to the rest of the immune system. These may be our earliest form of warning and defense. Injecting a tumor with BCG, glucan, or viscum (which we'll come to later) may be doing far more than just activating the macrophages locally. The dendritic cells may account for their powerful immunostimulatory effects.

Wheels Within Wheels

The level of organization in the immune cells is astonishing, especially when you stop to consider that much of it looks and behaves like primitive free-living amoebae. Indeed, Lynn Margulis, a biologist specializing in primordial organisms at Yale University, has suggested that our white blood cells might not be entirely ours, if we trace their evolutionary history back far enough. Small cells might simply have entered our forebears and stayed aboard to produce something new. If Margulis is right, strangers who, some billion years later, just happen to be working in our best interest colonized us. Or is it the other way around? Perhaps we are here merely to serve the macrophages' interests by providing a warm place to live, dead cells and cancers to eat, and by attracting bacteria and fungi and viruses to add variety to their diet—even packaging them for easy consumption. Such get-togethers seem to occur all the time. Termites, for example, are unable to digest cellulose and lignin, which make up the structural girders that give trees their woody texture and allow them to stand upright. Certain amoeba-like microbes to which most of the termites' digestive system has been turned over can digest these "girders." Without them the insects would starve to death. If an amoeba becoming part of an insect does not sound very dramatic, then consider that one amoeboid species *(Mixotricha para-doxa)* living in termites moves about on rows of undulating flagella that are actually bacteria harnessed to the surface of the cell. These bacteria bear a striking and possibly ancestral resemblance to the flagella that line the cells in the throat. Even more remarkable is the fact that the actual fermentation of cellulose is carried out, not by the amoeba, but by several types of bacteria living inside the *Mixotricha paradoxa.* It is, if you will, a commune of once independent and unrelated organisms now organized within a single protozoan, which is itself a part of a still larger organization.

Our macrophages and lymphocytes are like little animals crawling around inside of us, leading their own separate lives, yet under our direction in some odd way, serving to protect us from danger. Perhaps the most fascinating aspect of macrophage activity, or the activity of any of the immune system cells, is their ability to distinguish "self" from "nonself." Through the integrity of the immune system we remain separate from our environment. This inner image of "self-ness" or uniqueness somehow carries through to each defensive cell as it works to eliminate cancer cells that arise daily or virus particles as they penetrate from the outside world. The mechanisms by which this image of self is transmitted and carried out are still largely unknown. We do know that the mechanisms exist and, more important, that they are subject to change. Macrophages, for example, do not merely mope about hoping to bump against a bacterium or other source of food. They migrate from distant corners of the body, zero in on targets that they "know" are alien, and then destroy them.

More Immune Warriors

Like their macrophage cousins, the *neutrophils,* another immune system component, have a voracious appetite for foreign matter. However, they do not congregate in the spleen and liver, as do macrophages, but tend to remain in the blood, where they are far more numerous than macrophages. Their major role is to get rid of virus particles that have been attacked by antibodies. Like macrophages, neutrophils seem to migrate purposefully to trouble spots, particularly sites of antigen production. As part of the process of destroying foreign antigens, they release biochemicals into the bloodstream that trigger local inflammation and summon other defensive cells to action. If the inflammation lasts too long, however, it can lead to arthritis.

Eosinophils are yet other amoeboid immune cells like the macrophages and tend to show up at sites of allergic reactions and parasitic infections. They secrete histaminase and other enzymes, and appear to protect self-tissues from damaging immune elements, such as the inflammatory chemicals released by neutrophils. Eosinophils, moreover, are able to devour whatever originally caused the allergic reaction. These potent cells support the immune system's ability to kill cancer cells. This process can, however, cause an inflammatory response. When the inflammation is treated by prostaglandins, as seen in arthritis, they can also *inhibit the ability of the immune system to kill cancer cells.*

What can be done? Flaxseed oil and low-dose NSAIDs (nonsteroidal anti-inflammatory drugs, such as Indocin) are brought in to enhance the anticancer immune response, while the drug Tagamet in low doses can disinhibit the attack on the toxins. There is a blood test which can measure the support being given by the eosinophils called an Eosinophilic Cationic Protein (ECP) level. *Viscum* preparations discussed later (Iscucin and Iscar) can dramatically increase this immune function, as well as support the actions of the natural killer (NK) cells.

Another cell of the immune system, the *basophil*, has its surface coated with special antibodies called IgE. These antibodies actually function as receptors, sticking out like millions of tiny antennae. If a foreign antigen bumps against the cell and one of the cell's antennae happens to be an antibody against that toxin, the virus to which it belongs will bind to the antenna, much like a key fitted into a lock. This triggers a myriad of reactions within the basophil, including the release of such allergic mediators as histamine. These cause the blood vessels to dilate, quicken the rate at which blood courses through them, and allow neutrophils and eosinophils to get to the trouble spot very rapidly. These cells also seek out other copies of the antigen that set off the alarm. The intensity of the response is directly proportional to the number of basophils that encounter the same antigen. This important antiviral mechanism helps to protect us from cancer-promoting, if not initiating, viruses.

The *mast cell* is almost identical to the basophil except that it is located in the tissues and does not circulate in the blood. Mast cells are stationed wherever infectious agents from the outside are most likely to enter the body, particularly the linings of the respiratory and digestive tracts. What each of these cells has in common is a "personal," one-on-one relationship with the foreign element it is attacking.

YOUR IMMUNE CELLS

Biological Response Modifiers
Substances that influence the body's immune response; for instance, certain monosaccharides and polysaccharides (complex sugars) activate macrophages

Leukocytes
All white cells, any blood cell that contains a nucleus.

Lymphocytes
A special group of leukocytes that make up the bulk of the immune response.

Phagocytes
General category of scavenging cells which surround and engulf bacteria, viruses, and debris; appear as macrophages, granulocytes, and monocytes—Pacmen in action.

Macrophages
Cells that present antigens to T-cells, secrete monokines, and scavenge invaders.

Granulocytes
Cells that contain granules filled with chemicals to attack invaders.

Monocytes
These engulf and digest antigen particles.

B-Cells
Produced in the bone marrow, these cells make antibodies and are responsible for humoral immunity.

T-Cells
Produced in the bone marrow and maturing in the thymus gland and other lymphatic tissues, these recognize antibodies, regulate the actions of B-cells, secrete lymphokines (interferon, etc.), and lead to cell-mediated response.

B- and T-Cells to the Rescue

There are yet other elements in the immune system: the B and T lymphocytes. The lymphocytes are a family of cells that produce antibodies and direct most of the counterattack by the immune system. They do so magnificently if they are healthy and in one piece. Both B- and T-cells are produced in bone marrow. T-cells are so named because an essential stage in their development takes place in the *thymus* gland, which is perched behind the breastbone and above the heart.

After migrating from the bone marrow to the thymus, T-cells undergo differentiation as they seep down from the thymus's outer cortex toward its core. The differentiation or "training" process is apparently quite strenuous, for more than half of the T-cells will die and be absorbed by other cells before they can reenter the circulatory system. As the cells differentiate, new proteins appear on their surfaces. These are designated by numbers and referred to as "cluster determinants" related to the specialized function of each mature lymphocyte. It is from these numbered proteins that such names as *T-4 (or CD 4) lymphocyte*, which seem so mysterious in press reports about AIDS, are derived.

The T-cells have many tasks, including recognizing hundreds of millions of different antigens that may appear in the body. Because these must be continually sought out and destroyed to keep the blood clean, at any given moment, the thymus is preparing tens of millions of T-cells. Although only a few of these cells may recognize any single antigen (say, the antigen of a herpes-class virus like CMV, a universal cancer promoter), the collective scouting force is so vast and diversified that almost every possible type of antigen will be recognized.

The grand master of all T-cells is called the *helper T-cell,* or T-4 (CD4) *lymphocyte* (so designated because its surface is laced with protein no. 4). This lymphocyte carries no antibody weaponry, but directs other immune cells to attack (hence its name, "helper" T-cell). The T-4 cells fulfill the second immunologic imperative, which is to generate a *response.* According to the latest available evidence, the T-4 cell works like this: A macrophage, having dined on, say, a prostate cancer cell, secretes substances called *interleukin-1*

(IL-1) and IL-6 (mentioned earlier), which excite the T-4 cells. IL-1 also feeds back to the brain, which responds by raising the body's temperature, which further stimulates the immune system. Meanwhile, the excited T-4 cell releases lymphokine *interleukin-2* (IL-2), which stimulates other T-cells to grow and divide and also stimulates the *T-8 lymphocyte* (named after protein no. 8, a new protein that is made as the cell matures). The cytotoxic T-8 cell is a killer cell that can dissolve a hole into the side of a target cell (like a virally infected cell) and then move on, leaving the foreigner to "bleed to death," leaking goo into the surrounding tissues. This "goo" stimulates the dendritic cells. Potential targets of T-8 cells may include invading bacteria, the cells of transplanted organs, or the body's own cells if they are cancerous or virus-infected. In addition to activating the T-8 cells, T-4 cells secrete a protein messenger that causes B-cells to stop reproducing and to switch over to antibody production.

Once stimulated by the T-4 cells, millions of B-cells start making just one kind of antibody, tailor-made for a specific target. Other B-cells may transform into what are called *memory cells* whose job is to keep an antibody "blueprint" in wide circulation. If the offending organism should reappear, antibodies will strike as they fulfill the third immunologic imperative, which is to *remember.*

Antibodies themselves come in many different "flavors," able to match the "flavors" of antigens on the surfaces of cells and viruses. With the help of other proteins in the blood, they melt holes in the target cells. They simply bind to the viruses and produce antigen-antibody complexes large enough for neutrophils and macrophages to home in on. As all of these things are happening, the excited T-4 lymphocytes also produce a substance called *interferon,* which regulates the extent and speed with which all of the above activities proceed. Interferons (these come in different "flavors," too) are produced by a variety of other cells in response to the presence of a virus. The interferon "flavor" of cytokine simply keeps the process rolling along. Other flavors keep macrophages at the site of infection, where they clean up debris, including packages of antigen-antibody complexes. Interferons further stimulate B-cell antibody production, enhance T-8 cell killer activity, and greatly slow growth of the

DIAGRAM 1
Suggested Pathways for Biological Response Modifiers

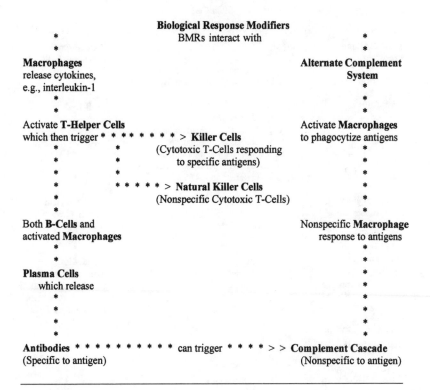

Biological Response Modifiers
BMRs interact with

Macrophages
release cytokines,
e.g., interleukin-1

**Alternate Complement
System**

Activate **T-Helper Cells**
which then trigger * * ** * * * * > **Killer Cells**
(Cytotoxic T-Cells responding
to specific antigens)

Activate **Macrophages**
to phagocytize antigens

* * * * * > **Natural Killer Cells**
(Nonspecific Cytotoxic T-Cells)

Both **B-Cells** and
activated **Macrophages**

Nonspecific **Macrophage**
response to antigens

Plasma Cells
which release

Antibodies * * * * * * * * * * can trigger * * * * > > **Complement Cascade**
(Specific to antigen)   (Nonspecific to antigen)

DIAGRAM 2
Development of Immunologically Active Cells

Stem Cells
(Source of all Leukocytes or white cells)

*   *

Thymus Gland   **Bone Marrow**
Precursor Cells   **Precursor Cells**
* * * * * * * * >   **Phagocytes**   *
*   (all scavenging/engulfing cells)   *
*   *   *
T-Cells   *   **B-Cells**
*   **Macrophages**   *
*   (engulf antigens; present antigens   *
*   to T-Cells for recognition; secrete   *
*   monokines, such as interleukin-1   *
*   to activate T-Helper cells; usually   *
*   found in tissues and RES system)   *
*   *   *
+ Antigen yield   *   + Antigen yield
T-Blasts   *   **Plasma Cells** and
*   *   enable Opsonization
*   *   *
*   *   *
T-Helper Cells   **Monocytes**   **Antibodies**
(regulate B-Cells,   (same role as Macrophages, but   (humoral immunity;
activate Macrophages)   circulate in the blood)   can also activate the
*   *   Complement system
&   *   and stimulate T-Cells)
*   *   *
T-Suppressor Cells   *   *
(regulate B-Cells)   *   *
*   *   *
*   *   *
Natural Killer Cells   **Granulocytes**   **Memory Cells**
(Cytotoxic T-Cells;   (contain cytotoxic granules;   (record past antigen
enhanced by interferon)   contribute to inflammation;   exposure)
*   includes neutrophils)

Mediators
(lymphokines, e.g.,
interferon, macrophage
activating factor MAF,
interleukin-2, -3, etc.)   This diagram understates the role of the
*   **Macrophages** in the control of general
Cellular Immunity   immune response. **Natural Killer Cells** play a
(cell-mediated response,   special role in attacking tumor cells.
e.g., Killer Cells, Graft Rejection)

body's own cells in the infected area. This is done to limit the number of new host cells available for infection and also to prevent the formation of tumors.

It all seems unbelievably complex, yet there is a wonderful feeling of simplicity underlying the whole scheme. Nature has pulled miracles from a disarmingly small bag of tricks, and the result is new cells that communicate with each other in extraordinarily precise ways by sending out little chemical warning beacons.

"Macrophage here . . . have located infection . . . working on it . . . secrete IL-1 . . . wake up, T-4 . . . T-4 here . . . working on it . . . secrete IL-2 . . . wake up, T-8."

Let the immune process go too far and the T-8 cytostatic cells will become "uncomfortable" because of an excess of certain biochemicals and antibodies in their surroundings. These will then chime in with alarm bells of their own, which are expressed as cytokines that suppress the activity of T-4 and B cells. It is a powerful checks-and-balances system.

Again, there *is* a simplicity to the whole scheme, and beauty, too, when we pause to consider that a thousand million years ago, when the brightest things on the planet were probably worms, simple creatures engulfed a whole lot of still simpler, amoeboid critters that have stayed on inside them, fusing with them, exchanging metabolic products and even DNA, yet remaining relatively unchanged ever since. Some of the amoeboids must have been parasites at first, but that kind of activity might have resulted in the eventual death of both amoeboid and host. Instead, those amoeboids that, by sheer chance, found themselves able to live inside the host, and by happy circumstance also preferred to eat incoming competitors rather than the flesh of the host, emerged suddenly into a world where a new way of living offered multiple advantages and, as such, became self-reinforcing. Look at the veins in your left hand, and think for a few seconds about the macrophages down there: cells that might originally have been foreign, yet now are orchestrated to defend self from non-self.

The Liver: "Immune Central"

The orchestration of the immune system and its tendency to destroy is tied, in part, to the liver. This organ is a hive of B-cell and macrophage activity. Let us first consider how some by-products of immune action are created. Viruses bound by B-cell-generated antigen-antibody complexes are adrift in the blood. Though rendered impotent by cages of antibodies, the dictates of human physiology are such that the only good virus is a dead virus (arguments about whether viruses are technically living or dead aside). The immune complexes are cleared from the body as blood flows through the liver's RES network, which, you may recall, is packed with macrophages (called Kupffer cells). Once activated, the helper T-cells begin to multiply, resulting in the release of *interleukin-2,* which in turn stimulates the production of still more helper T-cells and also *killer T-cells.* As their numbers increase, they release a substance called *B A growth factor,* which stimulates the production of B-cells and their differentiation into plasma cells—antibody factories (i.e., IgG, IgA, IgM, IgE, IgD). The antibodies bind to the virons and create large complexes that are easy prey for the macrophages, which can recognize the virus in this form and destroy it. The body cells that have been infested with the virons are attacked by the killer T-cells, which sacrifice these infected cells, hopefully before they can be turned into virus factories. The macrophages devour both the viruses and their cages, and they must devour them quickly.

Various components of the immune system can activate Amplification Loops to recruit even more immune response. This can be a powerful weapon against infections, but it can also lead to excessive responses, chronic inflammation, and immune system exhaustion. More is involved in improving immune function than merely stimulating immune responses. As discussed in the text, the entire system must be properly "fed" and modulated. Many antioxidants and plant compounds are used to help to control and direct immune responses to prevent exhaustion of the system and to control damage to surrounding tissues.

The longer the antigen-antibody complexes remain in circulation, the longer they will continue to gather antibodies. The cages will

DIAGRAM 3
Two Pathways of Complement Activation

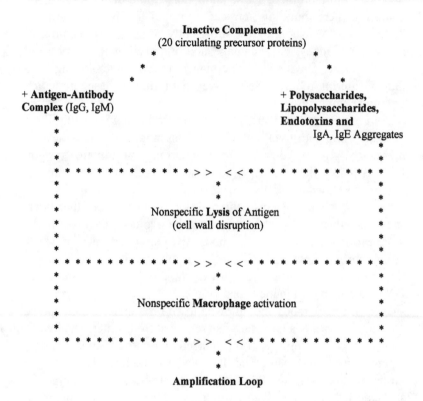

Inactive Complement
(20 circulating precursor proteins)

+ **Antigen-Antibody**
Complex (IgG, IgM)

+ **Polysaccharides,**
Lipopolysaccharides,
Endotoxins and
    IgA, IgE Aggregates

Nonspecific **Lysis** of Antigen
(cell wall disruption)

Nonspecific **Macrophage** activation

Amplification Loop

grow, doubling in size, and then doubling again. This continued growth has two effects, both bad. First, continued growth removes more antibodies from the blood. These antibodies would better serve us by being out there, building new cages around free-roaming viruses. Second, if a cage should grow sufficiently large, it may become deposited in a kidney, cause damage, and find itself unable to pass out with the urine. The result is a permanent microscopic blockage in a kidney filtering tubule. It is the liver that removes these circulating immune complexes.

And now you know one more reason for having a healthy liver. By supporting your liver with nutrients essential to it and by helping it to detoxify itself, you are in fact supporting your immune system. For this reason, if you happen to be suffering from a deep viral infection (like *Cytomegalovirus* or CMV, which the vast majority of us have latent in our systems), the addition of alcohol or other liver-stressing substances to the blood must be avoided. The liver is the largest organ (gland) in the body (if you overlook the skin). Weighing in at about 1.2 kilograms (3 pounds), it lies in the upper right portion of the abdomen, just below the diaphragm, and is divided in half by a ligament that connects it to the diaphragm. It is shaped into four lobes and, allowed to sit on a table, would spread out, something like a large jellyfish removed from water. The liver is quite soft, containing very little connective tissue, and in fact is only 4 percent less fluid than blood. It manages to hold its shape only by virtue of a thin capsule that completely surrounds it. Examples of substances that support your liver are two homeopathic/herbal medicines—*Choleodoron* and *Vitis* Comp.—and a supplement called Liver Formula.

Playing a role in virtually every aspect of the body's growth and maintenance, the liver is the only organ with a dual blood supply. A large blood vessel called the *portal vein* carries blood that has already passed through the capillary beds of the digestive tract. This blood is rich in nutrients, but relatively poor in oxygen. A second vessel, called the *hepatic artery,* pipes in fresh, well-oxygenated blood. The liver is tunneled through and through with canals, ducts, and vessels. These allow it easy access to pumped-in nutrients and rapid discharge of bile and other toxic products. The liver is the warmest and perhaps the most biochemically active organ in the body. It has an uncanny ability to regenerate itself and will grow back almost as good as new even if three quarters of it is cut out and tossed away. This regenerative ability was recognized thousands of years ago by the Greeks. According to mythology, the minor god Prometheus stole fire from the sun god Apollo and brought it to humankind. For this Zeus had him chained to a rock and every day sent an eagle to peck out his liver, which grew back to its full size every night. Once freed, Prometheus brought to people the art of healing. (It's no accident that the words *liver* and *life* bear a common linguistic root.)

Unfortunately, things don't always go as they are supposed to, or you probably wouldn't be reading this book. When we're stressed (expending more energy than our body can regenerate), things begin to falter. As the immune system becomes depleted, latent viruses that were being held in check reactivate. A frequent experience for people who later go on to develop cancer is to suffer from an attack of shingles (from the reactivation of the herpes-class, chicken pox virus) 3 to 30 months before the diagnosis of cancer. The virus didn't cause the cancer, but it did signal the crumbling of our defenses. If we take heed and take care, then things may not progress. However, more often than not, we don't and they do progress into lumps and bumps. Other herpes class viruses can reactivate, too, like EBV and CMV. These rogues, among other mischief, attack the B-cells. The result is that antibody production drops. I've observed that the T-4 cells, losing some of their T-8 cytostatic feedback, recruit more players and thus raise the T-4/T-8 ratio while slowing the maturation of T-cells into cytotoxic anticancer weapons. The longer this process goes on, the more immunologically naked we become. Soon, the population of natural killer cells begins to fall (which is why chronic fatigue syndrome was first referred to as the syndrome of low natural killer cells). With depleted resources and skewed pathways, our best shot for immune reconstitution and reactivation is from the back end up. When all else fails, the immune cells that we can best direct and reactivate are the natural killer cells.

Natural Killer Cells–The Cavalry in Action

Natural killer (NK) cells, which protect us from virally infected cells and cancer cells, are our last line of defense and largely function as independent contractors, as they don't need much antigen processing in order to do their jobs. Their name is based upon their innate ability to spontaneously and selectively attack and destroy a wide range of abnormal cells. NK cells mainly circulate in the blood and account for about 5 to 15 percent of the circulating lymphocytes. These cells can also be found in some tissues and organs. For example, they may represent up to 45 percent of the tissue infiltrating lymphocytes in the liver. They participate either directly or indirectly in multiple networks relating to the development, regulation, and communication within the immune system.

NK cells are capable of rapid responses by producing a variety of cytokines and other factors, substances involved in the interactions between immune and nonimmune cells. The NK cells seem to be able to coordinate their own counterattack even when the rest of the immune system is temporarily disabled.

NK cell stimulation is the first step toward revitalizing the immune system. Fortunately, much is known about this process. Since there is a well-documented inverse relationship between NK cell function and serious disease, including cancer recurrences, it is a process well worth understanding. Issues of toxicity and deficiency must be attended to first or we'll get nowhere. Having said this, let's wake them up!

Many different substances have been shown to increase NK cell function, but few of them seem to work reliably in the face of a damaged immune system. Of course, *sick* individuals are the ones who need to activate their NK cells, so they are the ones I'll focus on.

Two paramount issues govern NK cell activation. One concerns the "fuel" for the NK cells. The second concerns ways to increase the NK cell response for an effective counterattack. Let's start with "feeding" the NK cell. There are two major enzyme systems that the NK cells use to destroy their prey. If we don't have an adequate supply of these enzymes, then all of the stimulation in the world will be for naught.

The first enzyme that they use is "myeloperoxidase," which requires three important nutrients for normal functioning. First is iron. The use of iron for people with cancer is, of course, in a state of controversy at the moment. What seems to make sense is that iron be given when someone's blood level and iron stores (ferritin) are low. This is an all too common state of affairs for prostate cancer patients, especially when androgen blockers are being used, since testosterone stimulates the bone marrow and helps with anemia. Most men on these therapies find that anemia eventually becomes a serious problem. It can cause fatigue, shortness of breath, decreased stamina, and depression and lead to further immune dysfunction. A healthier diet and the use of supplements and homeopathic medicines can help these conditions.

The second essential nutrient is "a halide electron donor" such as iodine. Many years ago, Dr. Max Gerson added iodine to his therapeutic protocols and improved his results. Iodine also supports thyroid function, which is critical to immune, and specifically NK cell function. Iodine supplementation covered these two important bases. Today, iodine deficiency is less common with the widespread use of iodized salt. However, cancer patients whose symptoms are under great stress seem to need more.

Last, but definitely *not* least, this enzyme system requires vitamin C. Numerous studies and reports thoroughly establish that vitamin C enhances NK cytotoxicity by increasing the activity per cell, rather than the actual numbers of NK cells. Vitamin C is a good source of NK cell "fuel."

The other critical enzyme system for NK cell function is nitric oxide synthetase (NOS). When the NK cell releases nitric oxide, almost any cancer cell can be dissolved.

The metabolic stress of cancer also causes protein loss, leading to additional shrinking of the thymus gland and further compromising immune function. Supplements rich in the amino acid arginine, among other things, act as a natural precursor to growth hormone and will increase the size and activity of the thymus gland. Arginine also plays important roles in wound healing and protein synthesis. However, before you start eating grams of arginine, remember that it also serves as food for herpes class viruses, and we *don't* want to wake them up! So, take equal milligrams of lysine with the arginine to keep you out of trouble, and put you way ahead of the game.

Several sources of NK cell "fuel" are found in the world of herbs. In the whole herb form, one of the best seems to be astragalus. For millennia, this herb, also called Huang Ch'I, has been used in the Orient to correct "cold" and deficient diseases. If you need more than anecdotes, studies at the National Cancer Institute as well as other institutions have clearly documented its immune supportive effects. It has been shown to increase bone marrow growth and to reverse the gastrointestinal toxicity associated with chemotherapy. We're only just starting with the plant kingdom because in more purified forms we have some other powerful NK cell stimulants, too. But before we proceed, this is a good time to mention again that timing is everything! When building the foundation of our therapeutic strategy, if there is going to be a direct attack against the cancer in the form of radiation or surgery, then it is best done just after the start of immunotherapy. Radiation and surgery (currently, chemo really isn't a good option against prostate cancer) will result in the shedding of a lot of cancer antigens into the bloodstream. If this is done right when we're waking up the immune system, we seem to get a more powerful response against the cancer. (For other types of cancer, the timing of the circadian cycles also may be taken into consideration before giving chemotherapy.) Now back to the bugle call for the light brigade.

ANTIGEN ATTACK

1) Recognition
Macrophages and Dendritic cells "process" the offending antigens and sound the alarm.

2) Response
Classically: the T4 (helper) cells co-ordinate the counterattack
Alternatively: the NK cells can take care of some business by themselves

3) Memory
CD-23 and other special lymphocytes carry the torch (memory) for future reference

Herbal And Animal Therapies

Astragalus is a woody herb, one of many immunostimulants that come from the strong wood parts of plants. From the white larch tree (*Larix occidentalis*) and the laboratory comes a wonderful extract called *arabinogalactan*. When taken by mouth, it increases NK cell activity by activating the cytokine network. Arabinogalactan induces an increased release of gamma-interferon, alpha-tumor necrosis factor, IL-1, and IL-6, and seems to be an all around "good guy" as a powerful biological response modifier.

Currently, I am testing a whole new world of immunomodulators called "plant sterols" and "sterolins," which have potential for even better responses.

Working our way up the potency tree, so to speak, we next visit *Ukrain,* the trade name for a compound of extracted alkaloids from the herb *Chelidonium majus.* Many folks familiar with herbal lore know that if you have a wart and apply a drop or two of the yellow juice from a sprig of this herb, the wart will dissolve and disappear in a few days. Since the mid-seventies, the semisynthetic chelidonium extract has been successfully used for a number of different cancers, including prostate cancer. It has at least two useful and safe effects. First, when given in a "high dose" of 3 to 4 ampoules (little glass 5 cc bottles) IV twice per week, it specifically attacks cancer cells. Because it can become fluorescent under an ultraviolet light, within minutes of its administration it can be seen to selectively gather on the surface of cancer cells. When the concentration gets high enough, Ukrain kills these cells through mechanisms we don't yet fully understand. When given as a "low dose" of 1 ampoule IV per day, it stimulates NK cell activity and helps to normalize some aspects of immune balance. I have used it in combination with other agents with good success over the years.

However, the king of the herbal hill as a biological response modifier, NK cell stimulator, cancer cell inhibitor, stimulator of antibody-dependent cell-mediated cytotoxicity, and improver of the quality of life is mistletoe! In clinical use for over 70 years, it works best in comination with other therapies.

Moving into the animal kingdom, we have a couple of ways of specifically activating and directing the immune system. The first is by administering cytokines intravenously. Several protocols exist, which I use under different circumstances for my patients. Tumor Necrosis Factor-beta (Kinetrex™) can be given and is a potent anti-cancer drug. Pioneered by Dr. Ben Papermaster and in experimental use since the mid-seventies, it is now poised for FDA recognition. It has demonstrated both safety and efficacy.

Another protocol now in use employs low doses of genetically engineered INF-alpha and IL-2 and is quite helpful as part of a larger protocol with immune system disinhibitors, etc. On the other side of the coin, research has shown that if you remove some of the blocking proteins that cancers produce, through a process called double filter ultraphoresis, all of a sudden even a damaged and weakened immune system can fight back through the cytokine pathways that still function.

If you are a cancer patient, treatment protocols are available whereby your own blood and the tumor cells already circulating around in it are used to create, in the laboratory, your own cytokines (see Resource Section). These are then given back to you intravenously. This creates an extremely powerful immune stimulation and holds great promise. There is still some minor laboratory tweaking to be done, but all in all the use of these specific autologous (made from yourself) cytokines can be very helpful.

We have yet another way of directing an immune response that also can be life-saving. It involves a tiny capsule taken by mouth. This capsule is the result of over five decades of immunological work and research. It is a specially purified extract of the dialyzable fraction of bovine colostrum and milk (See Resource Section). Combined with the herbal NK cell fuel astragalus, its unique combination of transfer factors, defensins, and other low molecular weight immune supporting peptides it produces a "spreading effect" that strongly stimulates the natural killer cells and improves the functioning and balance of the immune system. These peptides are derived from the milk and colostrum of a standing herd of organically raised cows that were immunologically stimulated while pregnant. (It doesn't hurt them.) The milk and colostrum are then filtered, concentrated, and sterilized so that only the immunoregulatory peptides remain. This accomplishes a very similar pattern of immune reactivation and is an important part of the treatment strategy for *all* my patients. Once the immune system has been reactivated, the playing field is leveled so that it now becomes a race between the cancer and your immune system! This is a race that you can win!

Remember, cancer is caused as much by our bodily failings as by external carcinogens. As Dr. Rita Leroi, a principal clinical researcher in the use of mistletoe writes from the *Swiss Society for Cancer Research* in her paper "The Mistletoe Preparation Iscador in Clinical Use,"

On the other hand the environment exposes us to vast numbers of carcinogens, some with systemic and others with organ-specific actions. These only cause cancer in some subjects, however, i.e. not every chain smoker develops lung cancer. It therefore appears that both routes are involved in carcinogenesis—immunological failure and the carcinogenic effects of the environment.

This means that as physicians we must not limit ourselves to treating the physical body of the patient. We must insist on an improvement in environmental conditions, and we must also try and retrace in reverse order the gradual evolution of the disease, which went from the level of soul and spirit to that of the physical body, to put the patient on the road to genuine recovery. Anthroposophical medicine offers considerable potential for this. Apart from comprehensive medical treatment to regulate organic function in the liver, digestion, circulation, heart etc., physical therapy comprising the use of heat in various forms and a sensible diet, we also aim to consider the patient as an individual. Artistic therapies (painting, modeling, creative speech, colour therapy and curative eurythmy) address the soul-life, which in these patients has often grown rigid and tense and rather arid, aiming to activate creative faculties that in most people have become blocked or suppressed. We also enter into dialogue with patients to help them solve their personal problems and gain insight into their destiny and accordingly their illness. Patients often feel cancer to be an unjust punishment from God. They should learn however to see their illness as an opportunity for a change of mind and heart, allowing new impulses, new ideals to come alive within them. We endeavour to help patients to realise that their soul and spirit are an indestructible, God-given integral whole, and that they can grow inwardly because of their illness, even if it were to lead to disintegration of the physical body.

CHAPTER EIGHT

Hormones: Your "River of Life"

The balance of hormones in our body does more to foretell the future state of our health than any other parameter that we can now measure.
—Dr. Yulius Poplyansky, Director of the International
Foundation for Innovative Medicine

EXTRA! EXTRA! READ ALL ABOUT IT!!!

Stress Linked to Prostate Cancer

Sept. 27, 1999 (Ivanhoe Broadcast News)—A new study shows stress and social support are important influences in a man's risk for developing prostate cancer. Researchers at State University of New York at Stony Brook's medical school found men with high levels of stress and a lack of satisfying relationships with friends and family had higher levels of prostate specific antigen (PSA) in their blood, a marker for an increased risk of developing prostate cancer. The study appears in the September 1999 issue of *Health Psychology*. According to lead investigator Arthur A. Stone, Ph.D., their findings raise the possibility that a man's psychological state can have a direct impact on prostate disease. The study involved more than 300 men recruited through a prostate-screening program. The researchers tested their levels of PSA and had them report on their state of mind, including their level of stress and satisfaction of relationships. Based on the results, researchers calculated the risk of having an abnormal PSA was three times higher for men with high levels of stress. Likewise, men who had felt they had low levels of support from friends and family were twice as likely to have an abnormal PSA. Dr. Stone concluded it was unclear exactly how high stress and low social support lead to increased PSA levels, noting it was possible men in those situations engaged in unhealthy activities, such as drinking or eating poorly, that could increase their risk. However, he noted, "Other research has shown that stress, social support and other psychological factors can have more direct effects on the immune system and other physiological systems in the body."

There are many different types of cancers that your body can produce. Some of these malignancies are hormone sensitive. Prostate cancer is one of them. Hormones are special messenger molecules that are made by many different organs and tissues. From the very beginning of your life, your hormones have governed much of who you are biochemically. They have been with you from the moment you were conceived. They, along with your genes, define your physical expression, whether you are male or female, and how you look, feel, think, behave, age, and even whether or not you are healthy!

In a complex and intricate dance, your hormones circulate through your bloodstream carrying messages as simple as "time to go to sleep" and as profound as "it's time to make love." These powerful substances are found virtually everywhere in your body, in the tissues of your heart, brain, gastrointestinal tract, reproductive organs, kidneys, liver, and amazingly, even in your saliva and urine. (The presence of hormones in the urine is wonderfully useful from a testing perspective.) Hormones circulate throughout your bloodstream and coordinate much of what goes on within you. Each hormone has a specific job to do, a specific message to convey, yet hormones also work together affecting and communicating with each other in ways that are remarkable and, as of yet, like the immune system, often mysterious.

Hormones: Your Body's Messengers

A hormone is "a chemical substance which is produced in one location of the body and travels to another to convey, create, or generate a response." Most hormones begin their journey in your endocrine glands. The pituitary, thyroid, parathyroid, pineal, pancreas, and thymus glands as well as the adrenals, ovaries, and testes are all endocrine glands. Many other organs, the heart, for instance, produce and release hormones, but this isn't their main function. Together they make up your endocrine system, and for now, we are going to focus on those organs that are specifically endocrine glands and whose sole function is to produce hormones.

Like microscopic construction crews, biochemical substrates and enzymes come together in the endocrine system and are converted into various hormones. In many ways your endocrine system is one of the key cornerstones of your health. It manages, controls, and interacts with everything from your natural killer cell response to your levels of energy and stamina. The hormones regulate your blood sugar level, maintain the crucial balance among your body's electrolytes (important minerals like sodium, potassium, calcium, and magnesium) and enable you to build strong, healthy bones. Hormones largely determine how you mature and how slowly or quickly you age. Your endocrine system also helps you to digest and assimilate food, convert it into energy, and then use the energy to build strong muscles or burn fat. Sometimes things don't work out that way and some of us wind up a bit on the heavy side, but that's another story. Remarkably, your endocrine system not only monitors what is going on inside of you, it also monitors some of what is going on in the environment around you. It helps you to interpret what you see and experience, and then translates that experience into physical reactions in your body. This—hopefully—enables you to adapt to change and to cope with stresses of all kinds. Pheromones are a special type of hormone released into the air and are instrumental in the attraction that may develop when boy meets girl. . . .

Hormones tell your cells when to act. They are the spark that makes things happen. They turn things on and they turn things off, they turn things up and they turn them down. To everything there is a season, and our hormones keep track of the calendar. Your thyroid hormones regulate and monitor the rate of your metabolism and much of your immune response. If you have too much sugar (glucose) in your blood, the hormone insulin is secreted by the pancreas and helps to decrease it. If you have too much calcium in your blood, the parathyroid hormone calcitonin helps to lower it. Estrogen, testosterone, progesterone, and other sex hormones wake up your libido. DHEA, after it's converted, helps to create and maintain lean muscle mass. At night, the pineal hormone melatonin helps you to fall asleep, sets many of your circadian cycles, and supports many important immune functions. Sleep is critical for healing, especially the sleep before midnight, but it's the rising melatonin level during this time that does much of the work in helping to protect us from disease. Ideally, based upon the circadian cycles, to maximize the speed of healing that your body is capable of, you should be in bed sleeping by 9 P.M.! If you have any trouble with sleep, then taking melatonin is a good idea starting with 3 milligrams at bedtime. In some treatment strategies the dosing of melatonin can go as high as 50 milligrams! The list goes on. There is seemingly no end to the work your hormones can do.

You can think of your endocrine system and your hormones as your body's great gossips, exchanging information and greasing the wheels of progress. They are analogous in many ways to the more structurally rigid forms of your nervous system. In much the same way as a message is sent from one nerve to another, your endocrine system and its hormones are the means by which messages are sent over long distances in your body, mostly by way of the bloodstream. Information travels from your brain to your glands and organs; from your nervous system to your fingertips and the end of your nose. Many people think of the nervous system as the body's only internal communication network. In fact, if your body only had its nervous system to rely upon as a communication network you'd be sunk because the immune system, by way of the cytokine and dendritic cell networks and the endocrine system, conveys *much* more information than does your nervous system, just a bit slower. Nerves communicate messages using a kind of electrochemical relay system to move messages along from one nerve to another. For example, if you cut your finger, in order for your finger to send an SOS call for assistance, nerve endings have to be right there near the cut—and they are. That is why you flinch and say "ouch." The nerves in your finger pick up the injury message and send it immediately through your nervous system to your brain. Once your brain gets the message that you have an injury, it sends an alarm to your endocrine system while the immune system marshals its forces, so that your body's entire defenses go on red alert. Immediately, the hormone adrenalin is released into your bloodstream to activate your immune defenses and to give you the energy that you need to cope with your injury and to run for help if you have to. Another adrenal hormone, cortisol, a stress hormone, is later released to down-regulate the immune system and to help reduce any inflammation or pain that might arise because of the wound.

This is just a thumbnail sketch of some of what goes on and we'll come back to it again later because it's a critical piece for the healing process.

Your Information Superhighway

Let's take a closer look at how this hormonal information super-highway seems to work. First, an endocrine gland produces a hormone and releases it into your bloodstream with a specific message. The message is written in a kind of "chemical code." In order for the hormone to be able to deliver the message, it has to find cells that understand its code. These message-receiving cells have receptors and are found virtually everywhere in your body. They interpret the messages that the hormones were sent to deliver. In order to deliver its message, a hormone must bind with the appropriate receptor. Each hormone has a specific message to convey and specific places in your body to bring it to. Where a hormone goes and what it does when it gets there depend upon which receptor is its target and what that particular receptor is coded to interpret. For example, testosterone can bind with receptors in your brain and awaken your libido or combine with receptors in your skin where it can increase oil production. It can also combine with receptors in your immune system to increase the response of your natural killer cells that help to protect you from different severe or chronic diseases, including cancer. Or it can bind to a sensitive cancer cell and spur its growth. Each hormone has its own receptors, and even though an individual hormone may have different jobs to do in different locations in the body, it has to connect with one of its own receptors to create that response. In other words, a thyroid hormone molecule will not turn on a testosterone receptor or vice versa.

The relationship between hormones and their receptors is very specific. The way in which a hormone fits with its receptor is exact, like a key fitting into a lock or an antibody reacting with an antigen. Once the hormone binds with the receptor, it opens the "lock" and is transported into the nucleus ("brains") of the cell where the message gets decoded and the job the hormone has been sent to do begins. You can think of it in this way: Imagine that you are at the car dealership to buy a new car. You pick out a brand-new red Toyota sports car, fill out the papers, and give the salesman an arm and a leg (the standard price of any new car these days). In return, he hands you the key. When you step outside, you are faced with hundreds of Toyotas. Among them are Camrys and Corollas. At least twenty-five of them are red sports cars. Yet even though they all look alike, there is one unique thing about them, and it is in your hand. The key you are holding will only open the door of your new car and none of the others, or so hopes the dealer. Then again, nothing in this world is perfect, so you never know. As we've seen, sex-hormone binding-globulin (SHBG) can combine with estrogen or, more importantly, with xeno-estrogens from our environment, and stimulate an androgen receptor almost as well as testosterone can.

When a hormone binds with its receptor, one of two kinds of responses can result. The first one is immediate—it happens right away. The other response occurs over time. After a hormone has interacted with the appropriate receptor, its mission is accomplished. The hormone is no longer necessary. A team of enzymes then comes along to break it down. This process of hormone disassembly is also exact and specific. Hormone enzymes recognize the hormones they were designed to take apart and bypass the ones that they are not familiar with. The by-products that result from this breakdown process are called metabolites. Perhaps surprisingly, the breakdown of hormones and their elimination can be almost as important as some of the direct effects of the hormones themselves. Some metabolites are useful or even critical; others are essentially waste products that are sent to the liver to finish the disassembly and elimination process. How efficiently hormones are metabolized can also have a great impact on how well you feel. When it comes to hormones, your body knows just how much of each one it needs in order to function optimally. To regulate those amounts, your body relies on some very complex systems of checks and balances. Some hormone levels follow a regular, daily clock and rise and fall at about the same time each day. The sun typically sets these cycles. For example, the pineal gland releases melatonin into your system at about the same time every evening. Your melatonin level is higher at night and lower in the morning. If it were not, you would probably have trouble falling asleep because melatonin is chiefly responsible for telling your body when it is time to go to sleep. People who have difficulty waking up in the morning and feel sluggish until noontime may have abnormally increased production of melatonin during the morning hours when they are not supposed to be releasing this hormone. They should take an early morning walk outside without any glasses, which block ultraviolet rays. These help suppress this excess production.

Some hormones are released into your system automatically and predictably. They will always be produced at the same intervals. The interval can be every few minutes, as is true with testosterone, every few hours, or even every few weeks. Estrogen and progesterone function in this latter way, that is, on a monthly cycle. With synchronicity and regularity, hormones work together to manage your different metabolic cycles, including those of the reproductive system. Some hormones are released when the need arises, so to speak. Your endocrine system is constantly evaluating what is happening to you and deciding what you need in order to manage things. If you come down with the flu, your hormones are there to help you get well again. If you develop something more serious than the flu and have to take medications to get better, the hormones are there to help you adjust to the illness and to the impact of the medicines you're taking. If a loved one suddenly dies and you are left alone feeling frightened and isolated, your hormones are there to help you cope with the stress. During holidays and other times of celebration, if you eat and drink too much and play too hard, your hormones balance your blood sugar levels, monitor your water and fluid retention, and can boost your energy production to help keep you going. If you then decide to go on a diet and start exercising, your hormones are there to help you lose weight and build muscles.

The secretion of a hormone is determined by many different factors, including how much of it is already circulating in your bloodstream. In other words, hormones themselves, to a large extent, control their own secretion through feedback mechanisms.

This works much as a thermostat in your house does. If you set the thermostat at 70°, every time the temperature falls below 70° the heater turns on. When the temperature in the room reaches 70° again, the heater shuts itself off.

Similarly, if you do not have enough of a particular hormone in your system, its production increases. As the hormone in question rises closer to its optimum level, production slows down and even may stop altogether. If you go beyond the desired level and have too much of that hormone in your system, its production will stop lest it cause an imbalance and an illness.

Another important way the body controls hormone levels is through a binding process that renders the hormones inactive. Not all hormones are actually destined to deliver their messages. When hormones are released into your bloodstream, most of them—as high as 90–95 percent—bind to specific proteins. These are called "bound" hormones. They provide you with a kind of reservoir of circulating hormones that are inactive. They are unable to bind with receptors and create a response. The hormones that do not bind with these proteins—usually 1–10 percent—are left "free." These are the ones that can bind with your receptors and go to work right away. Free or bioavailable hormones are the only hormones that actually make something happen. This becomes important when we are interpreting and working with testosterone hormone tests or when we're looking at other substances such as prostate-specific antigen, and we need to measure the percentage that is free or bound.

As I've indicated, this system of checks and balances helps to control the amount of free hormone available to your receptors. For example, when your body produces testosterone, the specific protein called sex-hormone binding-globulin is produced and released from your liver. This protein inactivates most of your testosterone and assures that some of it will be taken out of circulation and held in reserve so that you will not have too much of it circulating. This also ensures that it will be readily available should an emergency or other appropriate situation arise.

Since testosterone has many powerful and positive effects on the immune function, during times of stress or injury more is needed to help your body cope so that a faster, more complete recovery will ensue. This mechanism for keeping "emergency" supplies available is very useful. The binding of these hormones also serves as a natural way for your body to protect receptors from overstimulation. This protective mechanism does not always succeed, as can be readily observed if you attend a boxing match or hockey game, places where testosterone levels are usually running rather high.

The protein binding also functions in another way. The protein can bind more tightly to some hormones than to others. This helps maintain a balance in the ratios between various hormones. For example, if you have 100 molecules of testosterone and 100 molecules of progesterone circulating in your bloodstream, the binding globulin will grab 98 of the progesterone molecules and only 90 of the testosterone molecules. Why? Because men need more testosterone freely circulating in their body than they need progesterone. Yet another way your hormone levels are regulated is through the dynamic interrelationships that hormones have with their specific receptors. Receptors, too, have built-in feedback mechanisms that control your body's sensitivity to the hormones. This kind of ensemble monitoring goes on among all of your sex hormones all of the time. Through a kind of syncopated rhythm, your hormones up-regulate and down-regulate each other to maintain the optimal balance that is your individual hormone profile.

Sex Hormones and Prostate Cancer

In the big picture of hormone production, one hormonal pattern dramatically affects your life: the rise and fall of your sex steroid hormones. As Dr. Yulius Poplyansky has written, "Sex steroid hormones, which include DHEA, progesterone, estrogen, and mighty testosterone, are the essence of your vitality, immunity, mental acuity, strength, and sexuality." Cortisol, while not technically a sex steroid hormone, also has an intimate relationship with these hormones. Men's bodies naturally produce the hormone progesterone, often used by women to balance estrogen in hormone replacement therapy. It can temper many of the effects of testosterone by helping your body decrease excess testosterone production. This can be useful therapeutically in cases of benign prostatic hypertrophy and in some cases of prostate cancer.

Testosterone is the primary "male" sex steroid hormone, or *androgen,* and plays important hormonal roles for men and women. Just as men's bodies produce small amounts of progesterone, women's bodies produce small amounts of testosterone in their ovaries and their adrenal glands. Until recently, it was believed that testosterone played a relatively small role in a woman's health. Even though women produce only 10% as much testosterone as men do, it is now believed to be vital to their health and well being as well. Recently dubbed "the hormone of desire," testosterone has grabbed a lot of attention because of its powerful effect on a woman's libido. But that is not all that testosterone does. Testosterone is an *anabolic* or "building" hormone. Anabolic hormones are like little carpenters; they help build things up metabolically. Specifically, it helps to build strong muscles, bones, and ligaments. When you exercise or experience any kind of stress, your body goes through a catabolic or breaking-down process. For example, during strenuous exercise, hormones, like cortisol, break down tissue and extract from it elements that can be used to generate the energy your body critically needs for stamina and endurance. In contrast, the anabolic hormones, like testosterone and DHEA, help the body to build itself back up and repair damage. These can be carefully monitored with laboratory testing, and we can assess testosterone levels for both free and bound forms. Supplements can be used to help regulate these levels for optimum performance and activity if they should be compromised due to a disease process.

However, testosterone's anabolic effects of helping to build tissue can have a profound negative effect. They can stimulate the growth of prostate cancer. Finding ways to balance the effect of testosterone with other hormones, or blocking the testosterone receptors, thus keeping the "message" from going through, becomes an important therapeutic consideration when dealing with prostate cancer.

Some hormones, however, can help fight prostate cancer by slowing it down and/or by stimulating the immune system. Two organs that produce such hormones are the thyroid and the adrenals.

The thyroid gland is located just above the base of the throat, and produces hormones that are indispensable for the normal growth and development of most of your body's tissues. Thyroid hormone secretion is regulated by thyroid stimulating hormone (TSH), produced and released from the pituitary gland at the bottom of your brain. Thyroid releasing hormone is produced in the hypothalamus of the brain and controls the secretion of TSH. The thyroid hormones are water insoluble, and thus require specific binding proteins to gain access into the cell and into the special receptors once inside. The thyroid hormones will then bind to their receptors on the nucleus and influence cell division. They also bind to special receptors on the mitochondria (small structures within the cell that are responsible for energy production). Once attached to the mitochondria, the thyroid hormones deliver a message that increases their activity and thus the energy available to the cell.

The NK cells, which are very sensitive to this effect, will then increase activity greatly as the mitochondria start pumping out their energy molecules. This explains why men who are low in thyroid complain of depression, coldness, fatigue, and trouble losing weight, among other problems. For over fifty years clinicians have noted that giving prostate cancer patients thyroid often helped them to do better. This along with iodine, a critical element for thyroid hormone production, was an important part of Dr. Max Gerson's cancer treatment protocol. With the introduction of iodized salt, fewer people are deficient in iodine, but testing for it may be useful if symptoms suggest a problem. Recent research by Dr. John Dommisse has demonstrated a more sensitive panel of tests to monitor for the otherwise sub-clinical hypothyroidism that can accompany any severe or chronic disease.

Another endocrine organ critical to the successful reactivation of the immune system is the adrenal glands. Situated atop the kidneys, the adrenals, however, present another very sharp double-edged sword. Many hormones and their receptors originally had been thought to be limited to one of three areas: the brain, the adrenals, or the immune system. It is now known that all three organs/systems can express these hormones and receptors. Medical research now links immune and neuroendocrine functions together and provides an understanding for the response of the pituitary and adrenal glands to infection and inflammation. Conversely, this relationship also does much to explain mind-body interactions and the suppression of the immune system in the face of emotional states such as depression and stress.

The Challenge of Stress

Houston . . . We have a problem.
—Apollo 13

All of us have experienced stress many, many times. Yet, when we try to describe what stress is, it is as difficult and elusive a definition as the meaning of life itself. "Stress" is more than just being uptight or having a bad day. It is a physiological imbalance that results in biochemical damage at a cellular level and eventually leads to dysfunction, debility, and disease. Said another way, stress occurs when the body is expending energy faster than it can be regenerated.

When the body is under stress, a whole new cascade of biochemical and physiological events occur in order to cope with the acute situation. This emergency system was originally created to help us deal with life-threatening situations such as the advance of a saber-toothed tiger or a forest fire, earthquake, or avalanche. The biological response was designed to be short-lived and to draw upon biochemical reserves even to the point of exhausting them for the greater purpose of the survival of the individual. When our stress response kicks in, one of three actions may take place. We will fight, flee, or freeze. The first two of these responses are useful in a primitive culture in which immediate life-threatening stress may occur. These two responses may still be useful on the seedier side of town where one may suddenly be held up at gunpoint. The fight-or-flight responses, you will notice, release physical tension, albeit they can also lead to exhaustion.

Because the stress response burns nutrients and reserves at a no-holds-barred pace, it was never designed for long-term use. An extended fight-or-flight response clearly would deplete the individual's reserves and reduce the ability to maintain normal functioning of the organs and systems. The ability to respond to a stressful situation and then recover from that stress and resume a normal physiology and biochemistry is referred to as an "adaptogenic response."

While we are no longer faced with saber-toothed tigers, we are faced with mortgage payments, birthdays, deadlines for book editors, crazy drivers and the like. While our primitive response to stress has remained unchanged, our complex civilization has created new pressures that test our ability to survive within it at a level of ease and comfort as we attempt to meet our needs and wants.

No longer can we deal with common day-to-day stresses of the world through mere physical exertion as we could have in the past when fleeing a charging tiger. Since our circumstances have changed and our biochemistry has not, our responses to these challenges are often inappropriate and damaging. Today we are faced with repetitive, persistent and recurrent stressful situations that did not exist just a few millennia ago.

When we find ourselves stuck in a stress response physiology, our nutrients are depleted, our defenses are exhausted, and toxins accumulate, often resulting in disease. Each of us has a different point at which our ability to adapt to stress leads to an unhealthy result. Many factors come into play: personality, behavior, lifestyle, exposure to environment chemicals, toxins, fumes, and our reserves of vitamins, nutrients, and substrates. Much stress is generated through an emotional response which is expressed—or worse yet, repressed. Aggression, impatience, anger, anxiety, and fear are all emotions that kindle the body's stress response. Eating a fast-food diet, drinking alcohol, smoking, taking drugs, etc., further contribute to our physical/biochemical strain. Eventually a breaking point is reached.

However, mental or emotional stress is largely what we perceive it to be. Some people may thrive in a particular situation at a particular level of arousal, while others find it terrifying and highly stressful. Not everyone is comfortable, like my wife is, with sky diving. For others, too little stimulus can be as stressful as too much. Psychodynamic stress only truly becomes harmful when we can no longer control our responses to it.

Shutting Off the Flow

In the fight-or-flight response, there is a huge expenditure of energy and a huge turnover of neurotransmitters, adrenaline, and biochemical substrates in order to support the metabolism of the musculoskeletal system. Blood is diverted to this system so as to effect the desired response. However, when the result of the stress response is to freeze, a different energy dynamic occurs. The energy flow is shut off, creating a situation where the person may be potentially able to produce a large amount of energy, but the energy that is produced is totally stagnant and not flowing in the way that will support activities.

For thousands of years Chinese physicians have referred to many conditions as resulting from *stagnant ch'i*. Ch'i refers to the life energy that flows throughout the body in defined (acupuncture) pathways. Its flow influences our breathing, digestion and the hormones, especially the adrenal hormones. When one "freezes" in response to stress, each of these pathways is impaired. If this stagnation refers to the overall energies of the body (as opposed to the energy of any particular organ), normal physical outlets are blocked and the emotions become "bottled up." One who is "frozen" in response to stress might be said to be "running on his neurotransmitters" (like many New Yorkers). The body is not fully running on the biochemical foundation that our systems were intended to run and function on, and this leads to a breakdown of the processes of repair and regeneration, which are biochemically based. Technically, we can almost always find abnormalities in the Liver Detox Panel, which shows us specific enzymes, how well they are working, or not, and the toxins that are backing up as a result of its sluggishness.

Ultimately, this imbalances the autonomic nervous system. This depletion of neurotransmitters, and thus its support of the immune system, is something that can easily, quantifiably and reproducibly be measured using either blood and/or saliva specimens. When such an individual has crashed, the knee-jerk response of conventional medicine is to view such a person who is experiencing a lack of energy and a sense of apathy as being "depressed," and to prescribe antidepressants (do you have any idea how much Prozac® is prescribed?) In reality, such an individual is not primarily depressed. Usually it is not just an emotional shutting down that the person is experiencing, but a biochemical depletion that the person is suffering from which, for all intents and purposes, will appear as a depression. This is why antidepressants are so freely given. In fact, many of these drugs will temporarily lift some of the symptoms and seem to be relieved for a period of time. This is a mere façade, and eventually the antidepressants will "wear off," the neurotransmitter levels will cross a critical threshold of depletion, and the person will again "relapse." It is not a real relapse; it is a wearing off of the drug effect because the foreign chemical can no longer synthetically support the depleted levels of neurotransmitters. In this situation, we have a person who then crashes to a level much lower than where he started. We also have the side effects of the drugs to contend with and the myriad of problems that they can cause biochemically. These include damage to various organs and systems that may have occurred from their use.

In my practice, one of the things that I have observed is that approximately 70 percent of the people who fill out my new patient questionnaire, as each new patient is asked to do, will report that, at a very early age, they went through a period of their life that they experienced as being abusive. This abuse led to a marked and prolonged stress response. The response of the patient as a child was usually to *freeze,* inasmuch as fighting back or trying to flee from an enraged adult typically had proved fruitless. I suspect that this learned response of freezing brought about a certain "shutdown" of their energy flow and created a survival mechanism of running on willpower and their central nervous system.

This response to stress, that of freezing or stasis, can lead to multisystem and multiorgan dysfunctions, including a failure of the immune system to maintain the boundaries of self and nonself. Research has shown that many of the receptor sites on T- and B-cells that lead to immune activation and control are the same receptors that activate that system in the central nervous system. Thus, neurotransmitters such as epinephrine, norepinephrine, dopamine, etc., not only affect the turning on the central nervous system but also affect the stimulation and response of the immune system. When the person is depleted of these neurotransmitters (as can be demonstrated by blood tests), not only does the function of their central nervous system falter (leading to insomnia, apathy, severe fatigue, trouble with memory, focus, concentration, and the like) but it also leads to an "apathy" and to a dysregulation of the immune system. One dysfunction leads to another.

With a disease as potentially devastating as prostate cancer, we must find out where all the energy went. First, we need to investigate the possibility of a biochemical failure, where the cells are not capable of producing the energy necessary to meet the requirements of the individual (as in a deficiency). This can occur, for example, in the case of a poisoning. Perhaps the clearest example is with cyanide poisoning, which involves an uncoupling of the electron transport systems (special energy generating pathways) within the cell. The Krebs energy cycle, the cell's primary energy cycle, is left running on a treadmill with no place to go and no way to get there. The result? Cellular metabolism fails and the individual dies. Other poisonings have less dramatic and immediate effects but are, in the long run, no less devastating.

The second possibility is that one or more organs or systems have been severely damaged and are draining energy at a very rapid pace as the body attempts to repair and regenerate the damaged tissues. This can be seen in someone recovering from any severe illness, such as pneumonia, hepatitis, heart attack, or stroke. The individual will experience severe fatigue, lethargy, and weakness, not because their cells are incapable of producing the energy, but because some major organ or system that has been injured is "hoarding and diverting" the energy that is produced for its own needs for repair and regeneration.

The third possibility is that the energy flow has been destroyed because of an excessive level of prolonged stress.

There is danger in any of these instances that vital organs and systems, such as the ever energy-hungry immune system, will be deprived of the levels of energy needed to sustain activities. Under low-energy conditions, the immune system will falter and allow chronic viruses to activate or reactivate. The consequence is shingles, or a reactivation of the universal cancer-promoting virus CMV, or something similar. As the effects of stress accumulate, the pituitary function begins to falter, the hormones that are secreted by the adrenal glands begin to decrease, and the normal circadian cycles begin to collapse. We see not only incorrect amounts of the various adrenal hormones being secreted at various times during the day, but also the timing of when they are excreted is incorrect. Many men wind up with reversed circadian cycles which, among other things, not only will aggravate the immune dysfunction but also will cause or greatly exacerbate other cyclic dysfunctions, such as in the sleep cycle (insomnia). A physician must support the patient's ability to produce energy, and help the patient to reconstruct his energy flow. Guided meditation and visualization have been shown to be of great help in this situation.

The adrenal glands are particularly important to our ability to respond to stress. In many ways, the adrenal hormones protect the brain from its own responses to excessive stress. Yet, paradoxically, the adrenal hormones can also participate in and often enhance the effects of stress. They can accelerate the damaging effects of long-term stress on the central nervous system.

In cancer patients, all these stressors must be identified and nullified. Toxins must be excreted, deficiencies must be corrected, infections must be treated, and psychodynamic stress must be healed. For example, given the common dynamic of past abuse and the related guilt, the patient through meditative insight and/or counseling must reach a point where he can "feel" in all of his cells and tissues a sense of forgiveness for the person or persons who committed acts against him in his past. Only by embodying a full sense of forgiveness will it be possible to stop the energy drain of these past injuries and allow the energy to be released and made available for healing.

This is not to say that if you are in a relationship that is currently abusive, you just turn the other cheek, so to speak, and let the abuses continue. It is not at all right to allow damage (stress) to continue to occur physically, emotionally, or spiritually at home or at work. Rather, one must first stand up to it. That doesn't mean that one necessarily fights fire with fire and goes postal against the person doing the abusing. Consider how Ghandi stood up to the wrongs of the British government in India and Martin Luther King transformed the consciousness of America. These great men were able to stand up to evil, not with guns in their hands, but with peace in their hearts as they carried their dream of a new humanity and a vision of a new and healthy society into current reality. One must stand up to one's stres-

---

DESTROYERS OF IMMUNE FUNCTION

1. Stress
2. Infection (T- and/or B-cell viruses)
3. Toxins
4. Deficiency(ies)
5. Trauma (radiation)

sors with whatever it takes to stop the abuse, to stop the injuries, to allow the healing to begin. If you don't draw the line, neither will your immune system.

Finding the Freedom to Heal

I once met a man named Tom with advanced prostate cancer who continued to smoke two packs a day although he claimed, through his rational mind, that he very much wanted to heal. When encouraged to stop smoking, he angrily responded that he could not. He had tried many times in the past and it was impossible for him to do so. When the issue of smoking was further explored, we found that he had been abused as a young boy, which had created a sense of vulnerability that he carried with him into adulthood. As he grew older, he found that he could, in a sense, put a smoke screen around himself and "protect" himself from those around him by smoking. He felt safer when he smoked, although he understood rationally that smoking was hastening his death.

In such a case, which is all too common in my experience, we, as always, have choices. One choice is to treat the prostate cancer the best way that we can, using drugs, radiation, surgery, nutritional medicines, homeopathics, acupuncture, and the like. However, a treatment in itself does not heal an illness; it only serves to ease the symptoms. The second option is to help the patient strive for a healing of the illness. This means that in addition to physiological and immunological support, we must try to help him through counseling, insight, and inspiration to reach a place of safety. The patient needs to attain a sense of knowing in and of himself who and what he is, a knowledge that can never be changed, regardless of what happens to him through external circumstances.

Such a transformation is truly healing. Through this peace of mind, the patient can then find forgiveness for himself and others that can correspondingly spread throughout his being and release his energy to be once again available for healing his disease. To be sure, this process is a Herculean task that requires the full attention of every cell, organ, and tissue. Sometimes this effort, even though it involves all his heart, soul, and might, may not be able to stop the onslaught of the cancer as his body may have passed the point of no return through the malnourishment and collapse of his immune system. Despite a physical failing, the patient may nevertheless heal as an individual by overcoming his energy blocks, by overcoming his fears, and in a very real way, by giving a new sense of purpose, meaning, and quality to his life. Such accomplishments are not undone even by death from cancer.

When one treats a disease process such as prostate cancer with drugs (narcotics, steroids, etc.), these can physically and spiritually dull the senses and one's search to seek and correct energy blocks. Often it is very difficult to try to simultaneously heal and treat an advanced, severe, and life-threatening disease. Often a choice needs to be made whether to treat the symptoms and thus try to prolong the *quantity* of life, or to try to heal the disease and go for a sense of purpose, meaning, and quality of life. The latter has been the more common and overwhelmingly successful course taken in my practice. Still, if it is not too late, and if one is lucky, one can stop and even reverse the physical signs and damages of the disease process.

Years ago, a scale was developed to try to rate the effect of stress on present and near future health. The stresses that were described ranged from a parking ticket to the death of a spouse. The more severe the stresses a person had suffered within six months, the higher the probability that he would come down with a severe or chronic disease within one year. Over the years, this stress scale has proved to be very helpful to me and further serves to underscore the critical need to identify and neutralize as many levels of stress as is possible. Research on Indian yogis has clearly demonstrated that the more focused a person is in the present moment, the higher the capacity for healing and regenerating the body.

Surprisingly high numbers of individuals who survived the bombing of Hiroshima were able to overcome the ravages of radiation poisoning. Over time, these individuals were able to repair the damages done to their digestive, central nervous, and immune systems, and were able to live a high quality of life for many decades after that severe insult to their systems. A corollary to this is the current research into the relationship of various genes to the development or risk of developing prostate cancer. Large groups of people may have a certain gene associated with an increased risk of a certain type of cancer. If one looks at people with a given type of cancer, such as prostate cancer, one may find that 75 percent of the people who have this cancer also have a particular gene. Nevertheless, when one looks at the larger population of people who have this gene, one may also discover that only 20 percent of these gene-bearers actually develop cancer. There are many unknown factors at play, and these factors are the ability of the individual to repair and regenerate damaged tissue through the health of the immune system and its ability to search for and destroy aberrant cells. This capacity to heal spontaneously depends upon the ability and access of the energy to flow normally through all of the energy centers of the body. The more one is able to walk along any street or path in the world with a focused, awareness and conscious approach, the better he can adapt to stress and prevent the onslaught of disease.

For the Physician
Useful laboratory tests:
Great Smokies—Liver Detox Panel: 1-800-522-4762.

From your local lab: TSH, FT3, and FT4.

CHAPTER NINE

Cell Death: A Time to Live and a Time to Die

The Lord is my strength and my shield; my heart trusteth in Him, and I am helped.

—Psalms 28:7

Case Study: Dr. Louis G. is a 59-year-old retired urologist. He had received brachytherapy followed by a radical retropubic prostatectomy and was on dual androgen blockade, but his PSA continued to rise. He changed his diet, started on my regular regimen, and stopped the antiandrogen drugs and started on Iscucin and a course of counseling. Over the initial six months of therapy, his PSA dropped from 22 to 0. He stayed on the supplements, added PC SPES to the regimen, and stopped the injections. His PSA remained less than 0.4 over the next three years that I followed him.

Commentary: The case of Dr. G. is another example of the ways in which treatment must be matched to the patient's particular needs. Androgen blockade was not helpful in his situation, but changes in diet and the use of special supplements succeeded where the drugs had failed. PC SPES was added at a point at which his PSA score already had dropped to near 0. The Iscucin injections clearly had reactivated his immune system's sense of the "otherness" of the cancer, but this likely is not the entire answer. It is possible to cause cancer cells to begin to normalize and it is possible to bring these cells to again observe their natural "death" cycle.

The Natural Life of Cells

Every normal cell in our body, as part of its genetic code, knows where it is supposed to live, what it is intended to do, how it supposed to divide, and when it is time to die. One of the big abnormalities of cancer cells is that they got the story all mixed up! New and evolving strategies are helping to put things right again by showing these cells the errors of their ways so that they once again die on cue. These strategies restore the preprogrammed mechanisms that control this process on a molecular, intracellular level. Programmed cell death, called *apoptosis*, is a normal process that is utilized to rid the body of unnecessary or damaged cells without inducing an inflammatory process. This "cellular suicide" is necessary for our normal growth and development.

Over the years, as we change, these systems normalize things at a cellular level. For example, maybe you've gone through a phase in your life when you've thought it best to exercise, and exercise you did! As a result of this activity, all kinds of cells increased in number in your body. Muscle cells in your arms, legs, and heart, for starters. New capillaries probably formed to feed these muscles and new skin cells had to grow to cover your now bulging biceps. Perhaps you know someone who, while jogging, tripped on a woodchuck hole and wound up in a cast. When that cast came off, what did that arm or leg look like? It was skinny! All that exercise for naught. Oh, well. . . .

How did it get skinny? With the limb immobilized for that long, signals were sent out and some of the cells shrank and some of that extra tissue died. This is apoptosis in action!

Except for the cells at the fracture site, the extra cells that died hadn't actually been injured. Injured cells die a different death from apoptosis and undergo characteristic changes called *necrosis*. Cells that had been mechanically injured (i.e., a splinter of wood), poisoned, or attacked by a virus lose some of their ability to control the passage of ions (like sodium and potassium) and water across their membranes. As a result, they swell, become leaky, and ooze their vital fluids into the surrounding tissue. This oozing goo is perceived as "danger" by the immune system's local garrison of dendritic cells, which then send out the alarm. Before you know it, you have a full-

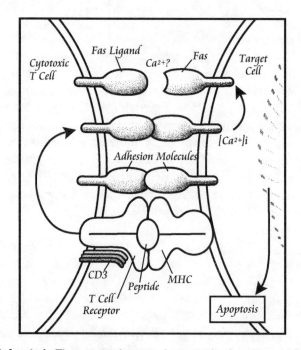

Figure 4. Apoptosis. These two pictures of apoptosis show our partial under-standing of this form of cell death. At the start of the process a Cytotoxic T-Cell adheres to its target. The T-Cell brings its active components to its sur-face and then releases these Granzymes and calcium ions to penetrate the target cell, where they disrupt that cell's DNA and cause its death from within.

blown inflammatory response: redness, pain, swelling, heat, and de-creased function in the affected area. The affected cells explode or shrivel up and are eaten and removed by macrophages and other mechanisms involved in the process of necrosis.

Not so when apoptosis is in play. When apoptosis has been trig-gered, special protease enzymes called "caspases" become activated. They are so named because these enzymes cleave proteins (mostly each other, as it turns out) at the points where the amino acid aspar-tic acid is found, hence the name: cysteinyl-aspartic acid proteases.

Once the apoptosis cascade has been set into motion, a number of things happen. The mitochondria shut down and break apart while the DNA in the nucleus is broken up into neat little membrane-

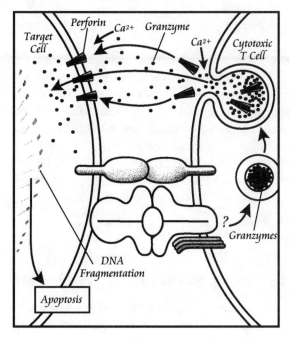

Figure 4.a

wrapped fragments, which are later eaten by nearby macrophages. These DNA fragments form a distinctive ladder pattern that neutralizes the genetic material within it. Perhaps, because the cell fragments are neatly wrapped and not spilling goo everyplace (disturbing the watchful dendritic cells), the inflammatory cascade is not triggered. One of the methods by which cytotoxic T-8 lymphocytes and NK cells kill virally infected cells is by releasing small signal molecules that induce apoptosis in the affected cell.

There are several known genetic sites that are critical to this apoptosis process. One of these, which I mentioned earlier, is p53. Normally a potent inducer of apoptosis, when there is a p53 genetic mutation, not only does it shirk its apoptosis duties but it can, in fact, become a cancer promoter. Research on intra-nuclear (inside the nucleus) antioxidants has demonstrated that in the normal, reduced (non-oxidized) form, p53 is a powerful ally. However, when it is in the damaged oxidized form, its shape changes and it acts as a cancer promoter. New types of antioxidants are being researched as one way of stabilizing p53 and restoring this normal pathway of apoptosis.

Many prostate cancers have been identified as having HPV oncogenes in them. The virus seems to either trigger or promote prostate adenocarcinoma (perhaps both), and thus is a critter to recon with. Fortunately, we have vitamin A (palmitate 10,000 IU/day) to help us. Vitamin A is one of the most common micronutrient deficiencies in the world today. Worldwide it's estimated that over 500,000 people become permanently blind because of its deficiency. It was the first micronutrient to be recognized for its anticancer properties and it is specifically known to help prevent HPV from damaging the p53 gene.

Returning Wayward Cells to the Fold

Since the science of apoptosis is still rather new, only a handful of studies have been done with natural agents. However, in those prostate studies several agents repeatedly shone like bright stars of hope. Among them were genistein, vitamin D_3, *Viscum album*, quercetin, and retinoic acid (vitamin A). Genistein, and isoflavone, is found in soybeans and is extracted through special processes to concentrate its activity. Another especially rich source of isoflavones is red clover.

Isoflavones are the subject of intense scientific scrutiny because of their anticancer influence on many human physiological processes at the systemic and cellular levels. They are sometimes referred to as bioflavonoids, and are commonly found in a variety of legumes, such as soy, and other plant sources.

Vitamin D_3 isn't really a vitamin, as we don't rely on outside sources to get it. Sunlight, which is the critical agent and more truly the "vitamin," acts upon our skin cells to convert cholesterol into vitamin D (cholecalciferol). Vitamin D has several anticancer effects. First, it has a protective effect upon various oncogenes and prevents them from getting turned on. Failing that, it works on the other end of the spectrum by sensitizing and/or inducing the cells into the apoptosis cycle.

Viscum album, an extract from mistletoe, also has especially powerful anticancer effects. Best used by injection, it stimulates the immune system, on the one hand, and induces apoptosis, on the other. It has many other wonderful anticancer effects as well.

At this point, there are believed to be as many as 20,000 different bioflavonoids. Bioflavonoids are made and used in plants to assist in the process of photosynthesis and to reduce the damaging effects from the sun. Some of the best sources of bioflavonoids are citrus fruit, berries, onions, green tea and bee pollen. One bioflavonoid, quercetin, has several important anticancer effects, one of which is to help induce apoptosis.

Last, but not least, is my friend and yours, vitamin A. Almost able to leap tall buildings in a single bound and stronger than a locomotive, at least on a cellular level, this vitamin is also the subject of much research and several books. Vitamin A has many wonderful properties. Now add to them the ability to help induce apoptosis.

New Strategies for Apoptosis

The strategy of inducing apoptosis can be greatly expanded and may even be employed systematically and rigorously through testing done at Rational Therapeutics Cancer Evaluation Center (see Appendix). Although only somewhat helpful for prostate cancer, by using a fresh biopsy of live cancer cells, this center can determine which treatment may be most effective for you based on measurements of cell apoptosis under controlled conditions. Dr. Nagourney, the founder and medical director of Rational Therapeutics, developed one method used at the center known as the EVA assay. The Rational Therapeutics breakthrough in non-proliferative assays is based on the scientific premise of apoptosis. With this new understanding, *we know that cancer cells do not grow too much, but instead, die too little!* The center's tests include many different drugs and some biological agents. In high doses some of these compounds constitute a chemotherapy, but in lower tissue-appropriate concentrations, they induce apoptosis. Research done at my alma mater, New York Medical College, and published in the *International Journal of Oncology* under the title, "Apoptosis and cell cycle effects induced by extracts of the Chinese herbal preparation PC

SPES" showed that PC SPES "modulates the cell's propensity to undergo apoptosis." One of the ways it seems to accomplish this was by down-regulating the expression of the bcl-2 gene, which protects the cell against apoptosis. By specifically suppressing this gene, PC SPES allows the cells to be normally sensitive to the apoptosis inducing effect of nitric oxide that is released against cancer cells by the natural killer cells and other components of the immune system. Thus, PC SPES creates a bridge to the anti-cancer actions of the immune system. In my experience, even in the common case of a weakened immune system, when the NK cells are stimulated and PC SPES is added to the regimen, "magic" can happen and cancers can stop and go into remission.

An even newer, but related strategy is to stimulate the activity of prodifferentiation. "Prodifferentiation" is the process whereby abnormal cancer cells, when in the right environment and given the right nutrients, will go on to complete the normal cell cycle, a cycle that culminates in apoptosis. Research in this area has thus far uncovered a few agents that fit the bill, and the search goes on. This may be the mechanism of action of a compound synthesized in the mid 1970s by the Greek physician H. Alivizatos. The metabolism of cancer cells is notoriously inefficient and mostly based upon anaerobic pathways. A number of research studies have demonstrated that if you take cancer cells and put them in a test tube with an energy (ATP) rich media, the cells will revert back to normal! Creating that energy rich environment in the body is easier said than done, but Dr. Alivizatos' product, now extensively marketed in Europe under the trade name of *Cellbal*, seems to make important inroads into doing just that. It also acts as a wonderful carrier solution for such items as the Viscum products discussed above.

Since enzymes are involved in prodifferentiation, regulatory pathways, like those responsible for the growth and development of cell types, are essentially cascades of chemical processes whose direction depends upon the relative concentrations and specific affinities of the substrates concerned. Few such pathways are intrinsically irreversible. The messenger hormones and peptides that govern invasion and metastasis in normal cells have normal and healthy functions. The environment in and around the cancer tissue—and the host response to it—to a large extent determines the resulting cell dynamics. This then creates the possibility for prodifferentiation and the continuing completion of the cell cycle in apoptosis. As the cells communicate and cycle more in harmony with the rest of your body, the miracle of a blessed remission can occur. This miracle has been documented clearly in many, many cases of cancer.

There are several important nutrients that help to promote remission. As described by Dr. Patrick Quillin in his book, *Beating Cancer with Nutrition*, niacin, CoQ-10, vitamin D_3, quercetin and genistein have been proven to be instrumental in bringing about remissions. The other nutrients were discussed above, but we cannot leave out niacin, also known as vitamin B_3, which is a very special substance. This vitamin exists in us in one of two forms, NAD or NADP. Both are powerful co-enzymes (substances that must be present for enzymes to work properly). The more than 150 enzymes involved in respiration and the transfer of electrons specifically require them. In other words they help make cellular energy. Without these enzymatic reactions, your cells would stop functioning and you would fall, crashing to the floor. Ouch!

Cellular energy, and a lot of it, is necessary for cellular differentiation so that the cells grow up normally and eventually cycle into apoptosis. Co-enzyme Q10 (CoQ-10) is essential for generating energy in all living things that use oxygen. Our cells produce their own supply of CoQ-10, but this capacity decreases with age and the stress of a severe or chronic disease. (Yes, prostate cancer counts.) Therefore, supplementary sources are quite important in helping to maintain a normal energy environment within us. CoQ-10 is found in fairly high concentrations in fish (especially sardines), some seeds and nuts, and in spinach. (Popeye was right!) It also acts as an antioxidant and stimulates macrophage activity, to boot.

For all of its wonderful effects (which are the subject of many a fine book), its activity in prodifferentiation is perhaps most important. Recent medical studies have shown that CoQ-10 can, in some cases, induce a "spontaneous remission" even in the face of an advanced cancer with metastasis to the liver!

Further research in the fields of apoptosis and prodifferentiation holds great promise for even more efficient strategies for intervening still earlier in the genesis of cancer. Other compounds have been tested that cause apoptosis and induce differentiation in prostate cancer cells, at least in test tubes. For instance, in earlier chapters it was pointed out that flower pollen/rye pollen extracts have been shown to benefit apoptosis and lycopene has been shown to improve differentiation. These and yet other substances await full clinical trials in human subjects. In the meantime, adding nutrients discussed in this chapter, which are known to stimulate apoptosis and prodifferentiation, is very helpful and is an important part of a successful and integrated treatment strategy.

PART THREE

On the Road to Healing

CHAPTER TEN

Integrative Oncology: Getting By with a Little Help from a F.R.I.E.N.D.

All human progress begins by asking a different question.

—Anthony Robbins

Questions are not signs of doubt as much as opportunities to crystallize what we know. They're a way of bringing knowledge and awareness to life.

—Bears Kaufman

Case Study: Alex G. is a 79-year-old retired contractor who three years ago was diagnosed with a non-Hodgkins lymphoma and 18 months ago was diagnosed with prostate cancer. As he was still receiving chemotherapy for his lymphoma, he opted for brachytherapy and a radical prostatectomy. He stopped the chemotherapy due to severe side effects and sought alternative care. He began my special supplement regimen, as well as homeopathic remedies by mouth. Dietary and other lifestyle changes were a challenge to him, but due to the persistence of his daughter, the changes were made. Now, six years later, both cancers remain in remission. He recently completed a house for his daughter on his property and reports that he "never felt better."

Commentary: Some individuals find that making changes in dietary and living patterns are very difficult. If possible, involve your family members, as did Alex G. You'll benefit from the extra support.

The Plan of Attack

As is true just about everywhere in life, the best outcomes occur when we have a plan. This is especially true when it comes to changing one's life. Being able to clearly focus one's thoughts without fear or panic is the first step in creating a new, healthful, Focused Response (FR) for your body to follow in its counterattack against the cancer.

With information gleaned from blood tests, counseling, and your doctor's experience, we then move into I, my personal favorite. This stands for Immune-modulation, the counterattack—help is on its way—the charge of the light brigade, starring the NK cells.

Next we come to E, for Endocrine-modulation. This includes everything from identifying and dealing with stress, to the actions of PC SPES and all its supportive friends that help shut down the cancer and nurture the immune system. When cancer patients are faced with a weakened and dysfunctional immune system, they need to find ways to starve the cancer, level the playing field, and buy time. It takes time to reassemble and rearm the immune troops. Until that has been done, taking advantage of the hormonal differences between normal and cancerous tissue is our best tactic.

N stands for Nutrition, the foundation for getting you out of trouble, and includes your diet and digestion, tackling deficiencies, and looking for any signs of anemia or cachexia and addressing them.

Finally, but really more at the beginning of the healing process, we come to the D, which stands for Detoxification. It's the sick/fluey/achy feeling that can occur as your liver starts to dump junk it has accumulated or when cancer cells start to die off. If we don't clear out the old stuff that started and supports the cancer's growth, then we're not going to get very far.

So, when you're working to stop cancer and you're looking for help, what you need is a little help from a F.R.I.E.N.D.

Since I'm a visual person, I have a special way to introduce you to your new F.R.I.E.N.D. As I mentioned earlier, the two questions I always try to keep in mind as I proceed with patients are: who is this man and why did he get this cancer now? Obviously, these questions will have many answers on many levels, but it's a good place to begin, and a treatment strategy will usually emerge. I've tried to organize many of the "right" questions from the point of view of my experience into a flow chart. (See Appendix O, "Algorithm of Diagnosis and Therapy.") Our next step is to explore that chart so that you can have an overview of how I systematically approach the treatment of prostate cancer.

The flow chart begins by artificially dividing the cancer from your defenses. By doing so, I ask, "What is your cancer trying to do?" I want to know about its p53 status (remember the soy isoflavones and the Cyto-Redoxin), and its cell cycle/DNA index information to know how aggressive or unstable it's likely to be. Of course, I want to know its androgen receptor status, which I may get clinically. All of this information comes together to tell me how to start starving out, slowing down, or otherwise disarming your cancer. Cancers with a low S phase (cycling rate) are more sensitive to pro-differentiation agents. Cancers with multiple cell lines, which aren't uncommon, become antiandrogen-insensitive faster. Here we also want to know if the cancer is metastatic. If so, Aredia and TNF-B given intravenously can be very helpful in slowing down the cancer and quickly stopping bone pain. Armed with this information, an individualized supplement strategy can be constructed which may look something like this to start:

PC SPES™	Take 2, 3 times per day.
Fermented soy drink	Take ½ bottle 2 times per day.
AIDECWE	Take 2, 3 times per day.
(Flaxseed oil combination)	Take 1 tablespoon 3 times per day.
Anti-oxidant forumla	Take 2, 3 times per day.

Add potassium and killer-cell support later. A triple antiandrogen blockade (Proscar™, Flutamide™, and Zoladex™) is very helpful, at least for a while, if the cancer is still androgen-sensitive and you're already on some blockade. This approach buys us time to figure out what else to do. Of course, your strategy may be a lot different depending on your cytopathology results. Still, the starting point for many patients looks very much like the above.

Now we get into the heart of the algorithm by asking, "Where are his defenses and counterattack?" This area of questioning is divided into three sections, as you might have guessed: biochemistry, endocrinology, and immunology. Remember the five things that can cause damage to your immune system so much that it becomes dysfunctional? Stress, infection, toxin, deficiency, and trauma? Well, we can dispense with trauma quickly inasmuch as the only kind of trauma that can directly damage your immune system is radiation. If you've been zapped, then you've been zapped, and strategies to deal with this situation are beyond the scope of this book. So let's look at the other four, starting with biochemistry.

As a recap, biochemistry deals with how your cells move things around, usually with the help of lots of enzymes. Good nutrients go in and bad toxins go out. I know it sounds simple, but it's amazing how often things get confused with a little help from our toxic environment and our empty calorie, fast food, gotta have it now, microwavable "cuisine." What's in that special sauce anyway? "$1.99— all you can eat!" Do you think if it really was food, they could afford to sell it for $1.99? By the way, did you know that, if you added up all of the chemicals in the human body, they're supposedly worth only $4.35? At that rate, if the fast food folks give you a pound and a half of chemicals for breakfast, they're still ahead of the game, even if it costs them a buck to wash, serve and clean the plate!

Speaking of toxins, do you have a history of exposure to pesticides, heavy metals (music notwithstanding), organic solvents, excessive (by definition more than I drink—which is virtually none) alcohol or coffee ingestion? Or how about drinking tap water from any number of wells and municipal water supplies across the country? If you answered yes to any of these, then you should probably have some functional detox testing done by your physician (see Resource Section).

The results of these tests can point to special nutrients that can specifically help support your liver enzyme detoxification systems. Other things that can help with detoxification are drinking at least eight 8-ounce glasses of purified water daily, massage therapy (to stimulate the movement of your lymphatics), an herbal cleanse, certain homeopathic medicines (choleodoron, etc.), and one of the oldies but goodies, the coffee enema.

Next, we have the issue of nutritional deficiencies. The RDI (Reference Daily Intake, which replaces the old RDA or recommended daily intake), is the minimum level of nutrition needed to prevent deficiency diseases like scurvy. Unfortunately, there is a *huge* difference between the level of nutrition needed to prevent a deficiency disease, and the level that is needed for optimal metabolic functioning, to support the detoxification of the liver, and to power up the immune system. Add to that the increase in nutrients needed to deal with stress, infection, or toxic exposures, and all of a sudden we have a new class of nutritional deficiency diseases called *cancer*.

While we're on the subject of relative deficiencies, let's start with things that can interfere with your absorption of nutrients. Top on the list are digestive tract infections. Be it viral, bacterial, or fungal, chronic infections cause damage to the sensitive micro-villi, the microscopic finger-like projections from the wall of your intestines that are responsible for the actual absorption of the nutrients. Indigestion, recurrent diarrhea, constipation, gas, bloating, and abdominal pains are all symptoms of an infection. Tests such as a G.I. Evaluation Panel™ or a Comprehensive Digestive Stool Analysis™ from Great Smokies can quickly discern the culprit so that countermeasures can be taken. Useful products include glutamine (to help increase the production of secretory IgA), soil-based organisms, and FOS (to help shift the intestinal environment), in some cases antibiotics and/or Diflucan™ (an anti-fungal), when indicated. All of these can help overcome the microscopic invasion. Chronic infections, and perhaps food allergies, can lead to the production of antibodies that can attack the gut wall and cause further damage. Such damage leads to inflammation of the gut. If we're trying to fortify the immune system, G-I tract problems must be corrected, or they will only worsen the more severe symtoms of nutritional deficiency, such as anemia and cachexia. How serious are anemia and cachexia? If left untreated, these can, in themselves, become lethal.

Compounding the problem of infection and our SAD diet, we have Father Time to contend with. As we age, enzyme production and the stomach's hydrochloric acid gradually decrease. Thus, even a good diet can lead to deficiencies simply because we can't break down and absorb things like we used to. Hence, enzymes are an important part of an anticancer strategy.

One nutritional relationship I do want to highlight is the balance between nitric oxide (NO) and lipid peroxides. As you will recall, NO is an important weapon used by our near and dear friends, the

Natural Killer cells to destroy cancer cells. However, as it dissolves the cancer cells, it also releases free radicals that can, in turn, damage normal tissues. The level of lipid peroxides in the bloodstream can approximately measure free radical generation. The trick is to drive the level of NO up with things like the amino acid arginine without pushing the level of lipid peroxides above the normal range. Lipid peroxide levels tend to be high just from the cancer process itself.

We can bring down the level of lipid peroxides with antioxidants and, if you have a history of a herpes class virus (shingles, mononucleosis, or herpes), you should take lysine to prevent the arginine from reactivating it. We certainly don't want to stir up the hornet's nest of herpes viruses.

In extreme cases of nutritional deficiency, you can wind up with the rapidly deteriorating condition of cachexia (extreme weight loss) described in a previous chapter. This *must* be addressed immediately! Working with a savvy gastroenterologist can be helpful, as can the advice of a knowledgeable naturopath or clinical biochemist. Hydrazine sulfate can be of help, as can Sun's Soup, an herbal "soup" studied at Harvard that showed its ability to help stop and reverse the process of cachexia and increase survival time all by itself. Having tried it myself, I can say it's not chocolate, but it almost tastes good.

The Mind-Body Connection

The endocrine system is our next stop in resurrecting your defenses. The issue here is one of stress and its medical counterpart, *psychoneuroimmunology (PNI)*. In a highly simplified nutshell, PNI views the immune system as capable of behaving like a sensory organ and therefore, able to be consciously controlled. It is the key to the mind-body connection. The powerful healing effects that occur when the mind is engaged in the battle against the cancer have been well documented for over thirty years in over 100 books and 9,000+ medical journal articles. Now it's time for you to recruit this resource and to command an ally.

One of the first researchers to begin quantifying the mind-body connection (the mutual effects that mind and body have on each other) was Dr. George Solomon, a psychiatrist at Mount Sinai School of Medicine in New York City. Using the knowledge that such major immunologic organs as the thymus gland and the lymph nodes were wrapped in nerve fibers, Solomon discovered during the 1960s that by electrically stimulating certain parts of an animal's brain, its ability to fight infection could be improved. By damaging those same parts, its immune function could be impaired. Solomon and many of his contemporaries began to suspect that feedback from the immune system might even affect the emotional and rational centers of the brain. This would explain, in part, why people get irritable when they are sick and why mental capacity often deteriorates in parallel with resistance to disease.

But no one was really paying attention in the 1960s. Doctors were too infatuated with technological wizardry and looking ahead to new drugs that were believed (a bit optimistically) to be capable of putting an end to all disease. Dr. Solomon laments, "I left the field of psychoneuroimmunology for ten years because no one would listen."

What Solomon at first dubbed as psychoimmunology fascinated the noted psychologist Robert Adler. He was convinced that herein lay a whole new dimension of medical science in which the nervous system played an intermediary role in immune response. He therefore inserted the prefix *neuro* into Solomon's term to create a true tongue twister—psychoneuroimmunology—that is usually shortened to "PNI."

Another leader in the PNI field, and a powerful patient advocate, is Dr. Bernie Siegel, retired oncology surgeon from Yale University. He combines visualization exercises with a healthy dose of common sense and wisdom. His goal is to help his patients gain perspective on their lives, and to know the peace of mind that results from it. "My message is peace of mind, not curing cancer or paralysis," says Dr. Siegel. "In achieving peace of mind, cancer may be healed and paralysis may disappear. These things may occur through peace of mind, which creates a healing environment in the body."

Modern medicine is predicated on the idea that one should try to prevent death. This is why, for example, the U.S. RDI (Reference Daily Intake) of vitamins is so low, as we mentioned earlier. The RDI is based upon the minimum amount of vitamins necessary to prevent common deficiency diseases and death from them, not the amount necessary to maintain optimum health (see supplement list at the end of this chapter). Any system of medicine based on preventing death rather than improving the quality of life (modern medicine being the first such system to adopt this approach in the history of humankind) is going to fail because, try as one might, no one can live forever. Instead of accepting perpetual failure, let us adopt a new goal or purpose for medical intervention: to live life with *passion* and *meaning!* Medical intervention then becomes a means to maximize the creative potential of each individual, to allow patients to fully explore and manifest their individuality, regardless of the limitations of their bodies.

To be happy and fulfilled; to have a sense of purpose; to accept, support, and love oneself, one's family, and one's neighbors; to be human: these constitute what it means to be *authentic*. Authenticity is another way of describing the healing path. To find purpose (the "why") in one's life is often the reward of an illness. When this realization hits home, suddenly you will find yourself standing, as if on a mountaintop, looking out over the telephone bills, the electric bills, and the ache in your hip, and seeing opportunity. You can, in a sense, recreate yourself. But to truly heal, you must first create a unique image of yourself, defining who and what you are and how you fit into your new expanded worldview.

"That is what PNI is all about," says Dr. Bernie Siegel. "Psychological and spiritual development are capable of reversing the disease process. In the figurative sense, it is as if all the destructive power that the disease unleashed is then redirected and channeled into self-discovery. Then, in turn, the cancer is attacked by a re-enlivened, purposeful immune system. The disease process becomes estranged and unnecessary. It is as though the victim had been reborn and rejects the old self and its disease. When a patient with a physical illness makes a thorough and positive personality change, the body's defenses, if still intact enough, may now eliminate the disease, which is not part of the new self." Such people are willing to do whatever it takes because they want to, in the words of the best-selling motivational author, Tony Robbins, "live with *passion!*"

What do *you* want? *Your mind is the key.* Everything else—vitamins, drugs, remedies, and herbs—can only help you stop the progression of the cancer. This is obviously a critical step, but you can *not* fully heal until, in your mind, you learn what you need to know about yourself and your purpose on this planet. You must truly believe that you can be well. Health may be defined as the full, positive, creative expression of yourself. Believe in the power of your disease, and you're lost. It's your choice. You can be in control.

If and when you realize this, then you will become a member of the limited and exclusive club that Dr. Bernie Siegel calls "exceptional patients." To help support these patients, Bernie founded an organization called ECaP (Exceptional Cancer Patients). You can learn more about them from Bernie at drbernie.com on the World Wide Web. If you have prostate cancer, you can further help yourself by joining their growing ranks to fight the good fight. These people, he says, "Manifest the will to live in its most potent form. They take charge of their lives even if they were never before able to, and they work hard to achieve health and peace of mind. They do not rely on doctors to take the initiative, but rather use them as members of a team, demanding the utmost in technique, resourcefulness, concern, open-mindedness, and love." Imagine this statement from an oncology surgeon!

This powerful belief system is the foundation underlying the biology of hope, to consciously choose and fight for one's right to live. Hopelessness, on the other hand, is just another belief and a way of choosing death. Which belief system do you think is going to keep you alive longer?

More Keys to Immune Support

Now that we got your juices flowing, if this book had an audio component with it, you would be hearing Wagner's *Ride of the Valkyries!* Let's turn our attention to immune-modulation, starting with the fifth agent that can cause immune dysfunction, infection. The first place to look is for the yeast *Candida albicans*. According to almost every medical textbook on mycology (the study of yeasts and fungi), Candida is an extremely common microorganism that will establish an infection anytime the opportunity presents itself. In virtually all men with cancer, because the immune system isn't working right, you will find Candida. Symptoms may include fatigue, foggy headedness, achiness, digestive symptoms of gas and bloating, and certain types of skin irritations. Usually this can be handled with simple diet modifications by avoiding things that yeast enjoys, like baked goods, sugar, alcohol, etc., as described by Dr. William Crook in *The Yeast Connection*. In severer cases, using Caprylic Plus™ (a neutraceutical) or Diflucan™ (a drug) can be very helpful and is usually well tolerated. In most cases, treatment is usually fairly short-lived because we are also working to reactivate the immune system, and as that task is accomplished, it will get down to business including killing Candida. The yeast is well worth paying attention to because as it grows, it produces and releases toxins into the blood that further suppress immune function and can thus prolong the whole treatment process. Furthermore, by eliminating it there will be an improvement in the quality of life.

The next critters we have to look for and, if we find them, aggressively eliminate, are specific viruses. As symptoms, physical exam, history, and laboratory studies dictate, HPV (human papilloma virus), HSV (herpes simplex virus), and other herpes class viruses, if present, must be controlled. Treatment can range from liquid nitrogen for genital warts to supplements that work against CMV, EBV, and HSV. Other approaches make use of antiviral drugs like Zovirax™ and Gancyclovir™. In extreme cases, an alternating low dose of the injected cytokines alpha-interferon and interleukin-2 can be life savers. This protocol includes a low dose of Indocin™ to help shift prostaglandin synthesis, Tagamet™ to help the immune system, and melatonin at a fairly high dose to help reset important circadian cycles, act as an antioxidant, and stimulate the immune system. This protocol also helps stimulate NK cell function while having a good antiviral effect. Research on bacteria that may stimulate or promote cancer is proceeding slowly and is currently focused on cell wall deficient bacteria. At this point the role that bacteria play in initiating and/or promoting cancer is controversial and extends back at least to the work of Dr. William B. Coley back at the turn of the 20th century. Unfortunately, much of the research that was performed in looking for a connection between cancer and bacteria was done decades before there was much knowledge about the immune system, let alone any immune function laboratory tests.

Thus, the explanations that were given back then now seem bizarre and have negatively biased further research in the field.

For example, while I was doing my fellowship at The Royal London Homeopathic Hospital, I heard about cancer treatments done decades ago from some of the old timers still teaching there and read firsthand accounts that went much as follows. In cases of terminal cancer, treatment may be given thusly: take a splinter of wood and stick it in cow dung and then poke it into the patients thigh. (This is *not* a joke, especially to those who had received it.) What would then occur was a monumental septic reaction and abscess formation, which if it didn't kill the hapless soul, may actually have resulted in a remission of the cancer. The explanation that followed described the belief that since a bacterium had caused the cancer, this treatment offered a type of homeopathic response—the doctrine that "like cures like"—which obviously accounts for the cure of those individuals who survived the sepsis. If we consider this from a more current perspective, we could demonstrate that fevers, up to a point, stimulate the immune system, as do the bacterial proteins themselves as a sort of crude and toxic vaccination. However, some *did* live to tell the tale, and had the scars to prove it. These days, I use Pneumovax™, a commercially available vaccine, in very low doses of 0.05 cc every other day as a small injection under the skin to help break anergy, i.e., the non-reactive state of the immune system present in most cancer patients. When the patient begins to respond, the injections stop. The Pneumovax™ not only generates a small local response, like a bee sting, but also results in the production of anti-A antibodies systemically. Prostate cancer produces proteins that have an A-like structure, so having the immune system make anti-A antibodies is an important step in the next phase of immune reactivation: breaking tolerance.

Tolerance occurs when the immune system doesn't react to the cancer, but allows the body to tolerate its presence. I use Pneumovax™ to not only wake up the immune system in general, but to point it in the right direction. There used to be a commercially available (any doctor could get it) vaccine called Staphage Lysate™ that worked even better than the Pneumovax™, but it was suddenly taken off the market without explanation. . . . The downside to Pneumovax™ is that you shouldn't use it if you have type A or AB blood, as the anti-A antibodies could cause problems for you. Instead, for these gentlemen, I use BCG™, also in the tiny doses as above, which will at least break anergy and get the show on the road. Breaking tolerance is vital in healing cancer.

Tops on my list to break tolerance is the extract of mistletoe (Viscum) called Iscucin (series H) or Iscar. Initially and in all but those cases of prostate cancer found very early, I give this daily, intravenously, in 50 cc of saline as a slow drip over an hour period. This treatment continues until the immune system is on its way to recovery. If a low-grade fever occurs (less than 100°), then I generally decrease the IVs to every other day or decrease the concentration of the Viscum. Of course, this is all supported by the diet, supplements, and other parts of the strategy that I discussed.

One of the more important supplements is AIDBCWE, as it specifically supports the response of the natural killer (NK) cells as they struggle to get back on their feet and launch the counterattack. Two capsules taken three times per day is a good start. When the immune system is back in full swing, I decrease the dose to one capsule taken three times per day. A natural killer cell support complex is another very important supplement, as it supplies much needed fuel and special enzymes that are useful to help maintain the counterattack.

It's important to look at the overall structure of the immune system, as this can give us important clues as to what went wrong to begin with. Toxic exposure tends to give us low T-cell and B-cell counts. Nutritional deficiencies usually show up with low levels of activated (HLA-DR and CD38) lymphocytes and both will result in low levels of NK cell function. T-cell viruses like HTLV 1, 2, and 3 (HIV) will strike first at the T-cells, deplete their numbers, and give us a significantly depressed T4/T8 ratio. As the T-cells falter, B-cell viruses will reactivate due to the lack of immune surveillance and decimate the populations of the B-cells, too. Needless to say, as immune function goes down, the risk of developing cancer goes up.

A very common scenario is the pattern of damage caused by the B-cell viruses EBV and CMV. Most of us are exposed to these viruses in childhood, and the initial infection usually just seems like a bad cold. If we're exposed later in life, then mononucleosis, the kissing disease, is the result. These B-cell, herpes-class viruses are put into a state of remission and held there by the strength and vigilance of the immune system. However, herpes-class viruses have two "interesting" characteristics. Number one, once you are exposed to them, they stay in your system forever. Number two, if you are under an excessive level of stress for a prolonged period of time, the virus(es) will reactivate. If they reactivate big-time, chronic fatigue syndrome will be the result. More commonly, they smolder and slowly chew up immune resources while reducing immune function. Specific strategies to deal with them are beyond the scope of this book, but are described in *Chronic Fatigue Syndrome: The Hidden Epidemic.* However, we can recognize their footprints as low levels of B-cells and later in an increased T4/T8 ratio, both findings reflecting the struggles of immune system to compensate for the effects of the viral assaults. One also finds a secondarily depressed level of NK cells and function as T-cells are diverted into T-4 lymphocytes to try and answer the cry from the macrophages and away from more advanced evolutionary steps into cytotoxic T-8s and NK cells. Hence, the name given years ago to chronic fatigue syndrome of the syndrome of low natural killer cells. In more severe cases of CMV reactivation, there is often a depression of T-cells as well. In this situation, immune system resources are being consumed and there likely is damage at the level of the bone marrow. At this point, both the cavalry and you need a little help from a F.R.I.E.N.D.

For further information see: immune-consultants.com.

CHAPTER ELEVEN

The Best Defense Is . . .

We judge of a man's wisdom by his hope, knowing that the perception of the inexhaustibleness of nature is an immortal youth.
—Ralph Waldo Emerson

Case Study: John P. is a 68-year-old retired telephone company repairman who was diagnosed with prostate cancer four years ago. He chose to have seed implantation, which seemed to work for about six months before his PSA started to go up again and his left hip began to hurt. A bone scan and X rays showed metastatic prostate cancer in his pelvis and left hip. He began treatment with Aredia, Iscucin, PC SPES, CoQ10, a super antioxidant, Moducare sterinol flaxseed oil, acupuncture, and a movement therapy called Feldenkreis. Over the next eight months, his PSA came down from 119 to 1.3. Repeated X-rays showed the hip lesion to be healing nicely, and John was again pain free.

Commentary: Time and time again, I have seen in my patients improvements that are not linked to standard forms of therapy. Movement therapy, meditation, guided imagery, counseling and other forms of treatment can sometimes produce surprising results. Remember the case of Ken V. in Chapter 2? Ken found that his cancer was in many ways a "gift" in that by getting treatment, including counseling, he opened to the richness of life he had been missing. Without his prostate cancer, he might not have made changes until it was too late.

One way of making sense of this is to conclude that all of us fit into a pattern larger than ourselves. Each of us has, on occasion, wondered what life is all about. The answer we give to this question goes a long way toward determining how we react to the world and its stresses. The answer also goes a long way toward determining how each patient's entire being is involved with his cancer.

Life is Ordered Energy

Of course, answers to the "meaning of life" question fill many a book. Nevertheless, we can look at life in a way that is helpful to the healing process. We can observe physiologically that life is the creative energy that orders the patterns of matter in accordance with its own rhythmic processes. Thus, the creation and maintenance of human life require a constant expenditure and *circulation* of energy on many different levels. Without this *movement* of energy, the activities of the cells lose their coherence with the whole organism and disease begins to manifest.

On a biochemical level, this occurs as a dysfunction of the Krebs cycle (the energy production cycle) of various cells, organs, and tissues. On a larger scale, without the hormonal control and the immunologic direction which the infusion of human life energy affords, cells and tissues tend to manufacture that which they are best at manufacturing—more cellular tissue. This is the predominate physiological activity which results in the disease of cancer. The physiological level of energetic activity is accessible both to acupuncture and to homeopathic medicines. I incorporate both of these into my practice for this reason.

This understanding of the necessity of the constant infusion and investment of energy for the maintenance and the cohesive function of the body goes back to the 1930s and the Nobel Prize-winning research of Dr. Otto Warburg. He discovered that if you take virtually any kind of cancer tissue and put it in a culture medium rich in the cellular currency of energy (adenosine triphosphate or ATP), the cancer cells will revert back to the near normal functioning of healthy cells because so many of their biochemical pathways are still working normally.

The infusion of human life energy must occur coherently and simultaneously on many different levels to have even the possibility of stabilizing, reversing and ultimately healing severe diseases. We can and do test for energetic functioning at my clinic all the time. On a physiological level, this is done through quantitative analysis of blood and bodily fluids in order to determine imbalances in the basic biochemical building blocks that the body needs in order to produce a "healthy" immune system and other cells. This may include amino acid analysis, fatty acid analysis, various enzyme studies, blood count, the analysis of different trace metals, immune functions, hormone levels, etc. Treatment on this level is then a logical extension of giving the person various nutrients, biochemical substrates and cofactors that his body is clearly either missing or deficient in for one reason or another. Furthermore, if the tests indicate a toxic pattern based upon exposure to petrochemicals, heavy metals, organophosphates or other toxic compounds, these substances must be dealt with through a process of neutralization, chelation (for example by combining with vitamin C) and excretion of the toxins so that the body can remove a major roadblock to the healing of cellular tissues.

When we are working on the physical level of biology, the logical progression of analysis, deduction, and supplementation is a clear progression toward restoring the fundamental materials needed for health. Analysis and quantification only go so far. This is a level of health restoration that is provable in that if someone is missing a particular factor and that factor is given, then the cellular tissues will function more normally, which can be quantified.

On the one hand, this is a linear progression in the dimension of earth time/space. On the other hand, however, we as human beings transcend the purely mechanical-logical-provable world of biochemistry. One has only to read accounts of some of the great yogis who under carefully controlled and reproducible conditions, have been able to transcend the seeming biological limitations of their body. To read such accounts or to see some of these experiments actually in progress is absolutely fascinating.

You can even have such an experience yourself using an inexpensive temperature biofeedback module that you can purchase at Radio Shack. You can directly experience how a change in your state of mind can have interesting, reproducible and provable effects on your body.

The simple experience of being able to raise your body temperature at will may be enough to confirm to your satisfaction the notion that you really are more than just the sum of biochemical processes. It may allow you to take the leap of faith into the spiritual energy dynamic that separates us human beings from our biological instincts and impulses. Health is to be viewed as more than just the absence of disease. It is a vital dynamic state that enables a person to thrive in and adapt to a wide range of environments and stresses while maintaining equanimity, humanity and normal biochemical functions. Our consciousness plays a necessary part in this dynamic. Moreover, from this perspective someone who "never gets sick" and then pops up with a prostate cancer obviously has not been totally healthy all these years. Some change at the level of mind and body always precedes illness.

When my young daughter gets a small cut on her finger and asks for a Band-Aid® to put on it, she does so with the full expectation that when the Band-Aid® is removed a couple of days later, the cut will have been "magically" healed. She is usually rewarded by her faith in her body's healing capacity. On a macroscopic level, healing appears to us as a miracle or as magic because all of the little elements that go into the repair of the damaged tissue, the removal of foreign material, and the fighting off and destruction of harmful bacteria happen in a microscopic world that is not directly accessible to our unaided eye or to our unaided experience of the world around us.

Nevertheless, her child's faith in the healing powers and magic of her body are an important ingredient when it comes to healing more severe diseases, a profound understanding that we can all learn from. Left to its own devices, the body tends toward health. Let me repeat that: left to its own devices, the body tends toward health. It is a self-righting system that tends toward stability and health if all other detrimental factors such as stress, deficiency, toxicity, etc. are neutralized and removed from the equation.

So then, why is it that people with severe and chronic disease don't spontaneously heal as a rule? The question one must then ask is where is this person's creative life energy going if not into the direction of healing? What is standing in the way of the magic of health?

The "magic," of course, is energy ordered to the needs of maintaining the integrity of our bodies. For energy to flow, there must be a "circuit" for it to flow through, whether we are talking about the simple circuit found in a flashlight or the more sophisticated energetic circuits found in living beings. The kind of circuits that we are looking at here are not just the electrical energetic circuits of the nervous system, but the subtler energy of the human field such as may be found throughout the acupuncture meridians. This energy is born out of our higher states of consciousness and flows in the direction of least resistance. Energy flows from an origin to a ground. This is the dynamic shared by all energy flow.

So, as a first step, what does it mean to create a "ground" for human energy flow? What does it mean to be "grounded?"

Groundedness is not a thing. Groundedness is an experience and a state of consciousness. Thus, like describing life itself, there can be no mechanical definitions, but rather a series of descriptions that characterize the experience of groundedness. It is a state of being focused and centered. It is a state wherein our consciousness can clearly be focused on a specific issue or event and not consumed in a sea of fleeting thoughts, moods, emotions and ideas. (Chaos diffuses energy.) Groundedness is a state of clearly knowing "who am I." It is a state of being mindful and present in the moment, in the here and now.

Groundedness might be experienced while playing volleyball or tennis just as the ball is speeding directly toward your head. In order to return the ball effectively, in order to score a point and not be injured by the experience, one must have a clear sense of purpose in that moment, a clear sense of being able to hit the ball in a certain way at a certain angle at a certain speed. This is a *focused response*. If you are thinking about other events or activities at that moment, then you will not be able to effectively return the ball.

Being able to clearly focus one's thoughts in the moment in a specific direction is one manifestation of groundedness. When we are constantly thinking about many other things and experiencing many different moods simultaneously, this chaos consumes little parcels of our conscious energy and our consciousness, thus diffusing it and preventing us from truly being focused, centered and grounded in the moment.

There are many things that consume our consciousness to the point of diffusing our energy and disabling it from helping us in the healing process. Some of the more common things that consume our consciousness are fear, worry, guilt and depression. These feelings stifle our creative healing flow of energy.

Passion, however, can move our energy and fuel our will so we can manifest our individuality and express it in the world around us. Passion is the movement of energy at a very high rate of speed in a short period of time. It gives us the opportunity to heal quickly. If I ask you "What do you do for fun?" I am really trying to discover your passions. If your answer is "nothing," as many men actually respond, this gives me more information about your prognosis than any blood test could ever give, and it isn't good. But if that were your answer, it's not too late to change . . . if you start NOW!

The Energy of Life

Where does the energy of life come from and how do we get more? This question has many levels and many answers. On a physiological basis, energy comes from eating vital foods. Foods that are grown organically, or better still, bio-dynamically, are "vital." Once your digestion is up to par, drinking fresh juice is an excellent strategy and an important part of a diet for recovery. Fresh, properly prepared juice is a major boost for recharging your biochemical batteries. (How else do you think the bunny does it?).

On a higher level, issues of purpose (knowing why you want something) and fulfillment (peace of mind) are important sources of the kind of energy that gets us out of bed in the morning and moves us through the day in a meaningful way. Higher still is the energy we have which comes from truly knowing ourselves (enlightenment) and knowing how to reach out and tap into the energy resources that are in and around us. For example, if you are having a tough day and are not feeling well, having enough perspective to understand your state and knowing which special friend to call or what movie to go see or what creative project to work on in the garage can shift the way you feel and imbue you with a new charge of energy. Your state of consciousness dictates your experience of life. As you will shortly learn, your state of consciousness also plays a key role in determining the outcome of your battle with cancer.

But where does our consciousness begin?

To that question we can ultimately only answer with the word *intention*. Intention is the desire to create something or bring something into reality that does not yet exist. In the clarity and peacefulness of your consciousness, you experience the desire for potential before it is born. You have a desire for air before it becomes breath, a desire for thought before it becomes an idea, the desire for sound before it is heard and a desire for an image before it can be seen. Just as you were born of God's intention, healing that comes through you is born from your intention. Before you can embark upon a new journey, whether through your mind or in your body or spirit, there needs to be intention. Before an idea, a word or an action occurs, all aspects of who you are call to you and ask what is your intention. When you know your intention, your spirit knows its purpose. Your mind, heart and will define their goals and your body responds accordingly.

With clear, pure, focused intention, healing can quickly occur from any illness if it is not advanced to the point of the total dissolution of organs and tissues. Such healing requires the clear and congruent alignment of all of the resources of your body, mind and spirit. When you accept the reality of the illness, yet avoid attaching to its dominating all parts of your life, you can make peace with the suffering and go on. Making peace with adversity is necessary for men suffering from prostate cancer. A disease that short-circuits your life plans, changes your lifestyle and creates havoc in your mind can also serve to bring a semblance of meaning to your life. When you accept yourself and the blistering storm of emotions and frustrations as part of life, you are then free to move beyond the disease and healing can occur.

Your attitude lays the foundation for the possibility for healing to unfold—or not. When dealing with this potentially lethal disease, the best attitude to hold is one of gratitude: gratitude for the life you still have to live and the love you have yet to share. To again quote author Tony Robbins, "gratitude antidotes fear." At first, for many such a thought seems ludicrous, what with all the discomforts, compromises and losses that prostate cancer can bring with it. So start small, perhaps by focusing upon a photograph of a grandchild, the beauty of a crystal that you keep in your pocket or even just looking up at a magnificent cloud formation or sunset, something that will begin to stir in your heart. Your body will relax, stress will subside and a new perspective on life can begin to take root. Holding this focus will help you maintain positive expectations for the future which will further serve to support your immune system and, strengthen your defenses.

Attitude is often affected by conscious and unconscious guilt, which keeps our energy rooted in the past and unavailable for healing us now. For centuries the Catholic Church has been using a system of confession to unburden the spirit and bring one closer to God, wholeness and healing. Modern medicine has begun to research this healing power and apply it in some very powerful and dynamic ways.

One of the pioneers in this field, known as *"disclosure,"* is Dr. James A. Around-Thomas, who worked out a reproducible methodology for applying this newest of "sciences." He refers to his work as Integrative Behavioral Oncology and describes it in detail in his forthcoming book. The bottom line is that whatever happened in the past has to be released from holding you back now. You need all of the energy that you can find to heal from prostate cancer. Forgiveness is a key to healing, so start with yourself!!

This is *not* to say that if someone does you wrong that you should just accept it and say, "thank you." Heck NO! That would only weaken your defenses by failing to set an example, if you will, for your immune system of what boundaries are all about. To re-enliven your immune system on an energetic level requires an opening of your heart, on the one hand, to allow energy to flow, and the establishment of strict no-nonsense boundaries, on the other hand, so that "self from non-self" become easily recognized domains. You must ruthlessly defend against intrusions into the safe, healing space that you create for yourself. For example, turn off the telephone, except for a specific time each day, so as to avoid unimportant intrusions into the new healing daily routine that you are creating for yourself. After all, what's really important, staying as long as possible in a stress-less, mindful state or answering the phone and talking to some computer that's trying to sell you a magazine subscription to God-knows-what?

For many men this shift occurs when they embrace a religious or spiritual path; for others, counseling is the key that unlocks the doorway to recovery. In any case, I've never seen anyone attain a long-term recovery from cancer without experiencing such a shift. I've met too many ministers, rabbis and mechanics who had forgotten the second part of the formula for immune empowerment: the need to proclaim their right to exist! These forces of intention (embracing both openness and necessary boundaries) balance each other into *The Path of the Peaceful Warrior* and invoke a new paradigm of self for your physiology to emulate, thus stimulating immune function. Of course, we must feed and detoxify your system, but as the saying goes, "man does not live by bread alone." Unfortunately, in our society, it is the subtler elements of the healing process (for example, stress reduction) that are often discounted or overlooked to the detriment of the outcome that we want. As Norman Cousins pointed out:

> There is a healing biological response to hope. . . . Concern over "false hopes" tends to ignore the far more prevalent problem caused by "false fears." People tell me not to offer hope unless I know hope to be real, but I don't have the power not to respond to an outstretched hand. . . . I'm not sure anyone knows enough to deny hope. I have seen too many cases, these past ten years, when death predictions were delivered from high professional station only to be gloriously refuted by patients for reasons having less to do with tangible biology than the human spirit, admittedly a vague term but one that may well be the greatest force of all within the human arsenal.

Cancer is not really a part of the human organism. Instead, it represents a rebellion of the cells against us, it is a selfish parasite. A tumor can only occur if the growth processes of the cells proceed unchecked. Cancer is a result of the disruption of your body's growth forces as well as a failure of the communication and integration of your individual identity. Therefore, cancer is a dynamic maladaptive *process* that originates within normal tissues, is constantly in evolution and is potentially reversible. It is not a discrete morphological entity.

The increase of the incidence, diversity and accelerated progression of cancers in *immuno-suppressed* and *depressed* patients is well documented. Mind and body work together. This perspective is critical for understanding the integrative strategies that I use. These strategies can stop and reverse the disease process and can prevent its recurrence, as described elsewhere in the book. The bottom line is that the "host" response is critical; it ultimately determines the long-term outcome. The 10s of thousands of books and research papers published in the field of oncology, if nothing else, have clearly demonstrated that the growth rates of cancer cells are variable and depend upon the regulatory balance within themselves and in relationship to the "host" that they are invading. This unbalanced environment is potentially reversible and may lead to the "functional cure" of long-term remission. This "cure" can last the rest of your natural life.

I have a name for my particular mind-body approach. I call it the **S**piritual, **P**hysiological, **A**ttitudinal, **M**ilieu approach, or **SPAM** for short. It may be a tough concept to swallow, but it can keep you alive and is the foundation of your defenses. It determines the results of the interaction between the cancer and yourself. In contrast, treatments solely based upon drug therapies designed only to induce a remission by attacking the cancer as a local phenomenon do not necessarily bring about cures. In the inspired article, "Shifting the Cancer Paradigm: Must We Kill to Cure?" an editorial appearing in the *Journal of Clinical Oncology*, the editors wrote:

> There is now ample data showing that remission does not predict cure, e.g., the failure of adjuvant therapies to flatten survival or disease-free survival curves, the incidence of relapse after long periods of remission, and the development of secondary or transformed (androgen resistant) malignancies. Viewed from the opposite perspective, a persistent tumor does not necessarily predict morbidity or mortality.

The healing process can only proceed at a deliberate pace, at a slow walk, perhaps, but not at a fast jog. There are too many bases to cover, bridges to mend and defenses to refortify. Yet, by steadily re-building the body's defenses and consciously focusing on the tasks at hand to create the outcome that you want (the "what"), while clearly aligning yourself to your purpose (the "why") for doing so, you someday may find yourself standing up to say of cancer, "this too shall pass," and it will.

Epilogue

Begin difficult things
While they are easy,

Do great things
When they are small,

The difficult things of the world
Must once have been easy;

The great things
Must once have been small. . . .

A thousand mile journey
Begins with
A single step.

—Lao Tse

The act of taking that first step is born from great courage. Courage in turn is founded upon the hope for the outcome that you want and the faith that you can achieve it. Hope can free the ill from despair and help achieve a good quality of life and a purpose for living. Hope, transformed by the will of the human spirit, can sustain life, even under the most difficult of circumstances. Life is the greatest prize and it takes on ultimate value when we suddenly discover how tentative and fragile it can be. The essential art of healing and living is to respect and savor its preciousness from the smallest frog to the entire planet Earth. I pray that you find the courage to take that first step toward reclaiming your life and finding peace.

—Jesse A. Stoff, M.D.
dr-stoff.com

Appendices

The Algorithm—Helping Us Ask the Right Questions

When faced with a challenging medical situation, i.e., someone with prostate cancer, there isn't only one "right" place to start the therapeutic process. Physicians keep asking questions both of the patient and the laboratory (lab tests) until they find a place that's comfortable, reasonable, and familiar to dig in and begin fighting back. Like a meditative maze, there may be several good starting places but, ultimately, if you're on the right track, they all have a common final ending place known as remission.

Throughout this book we have asked many such questions, just as any treatment team that you are working with should do. From a book you can never get the answer of where the "best" place for YOU to begin is. That is something for you and your team to decide. When faced with several possible treatment choices, one way that physicians decide which way to precede is to boil the whole thing down into a simpler graphic representation called an algorithm.

An algorithm gives us a more linear way of asking "the right" questions and correlating them to reasonable therapeutic choices. On the following pages are algorithms that summarize the key points that we have made in the course of this text. Another way to think of them is as a cookbook. Cookbooks are useful because they can focus the decision-making process and serve as teaching tools, but they are limited by their very nature of being two-dimensional pre-programmed, inflexible crutches. Short-order cooks follow a cookbook. Master chefs follow their intuition guided by their experience and inspirations. Short-order cooks treat cancer, master chefs treat people.

Look for a master chef who can use a cookbook but who isn't limited by it. The award-winning recipe that he or she can make for you is called a remission, and is best served with joy and passion!

PROSTATE CANCER

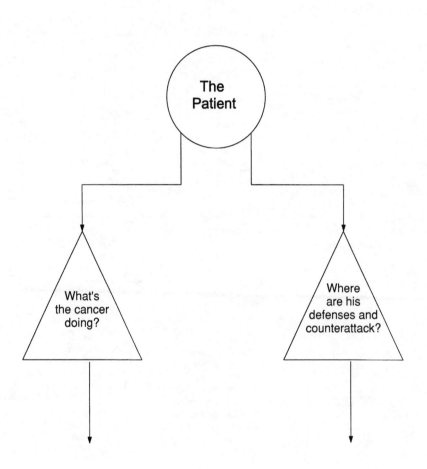

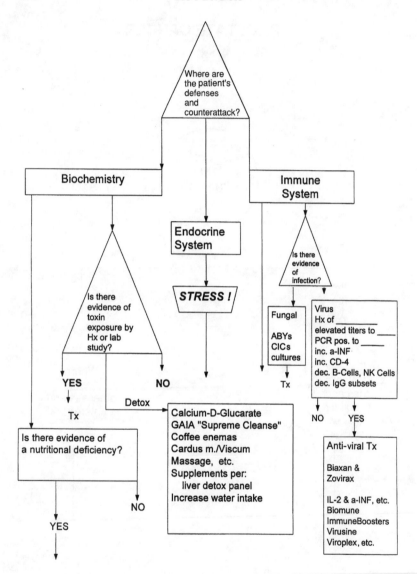

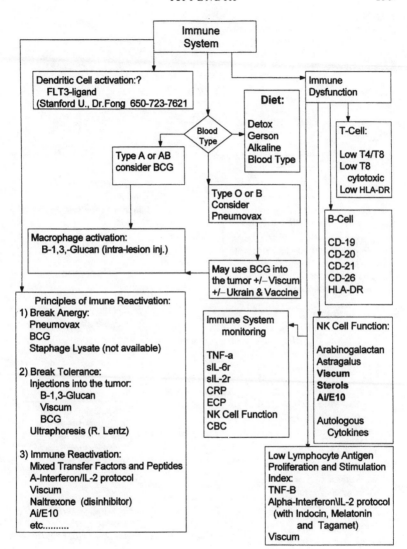

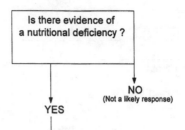

Is there evidence of
a nutritional deficiency ?

YES

NO
(Not a likely response)

ABSOLUTE DEFICIENCIES
(dietary)
Vit A
Vit D
Vit A/D ratio
Se
NO (Arginine use "NK Daily")
Lipid Peroxides (need anti-oxidants)
B6
Lignans from Flaxseed oil
Eicosapentaenoic acid (EPA)

Anemia

Amino chelated iron (Hemecomplex)
Pulsatilla
Alkyrol

Additional
Support

Enzymes****
Vit C
Niacin or Inositol-Niacinate
CoQ 10
Calmodulin
Maitake -D

Cachexia

Vivonex Plus
Hydrazine Sulfate
Megace
Sun Soup

RELATIVE DEFICIENCIES
from:
G. I. DAMAGE
  increased CD-71
  G.I. permeability index
AUTOIMMUNE PROBLEMS
  Anti-Parietal Cell ABYs
  Anti-Intrinsic Factor ABYs
  Anti-Gliadin ABYs
  Anti-Chief Cell ABYs
CHRONIC/SUBACUTE INFECTIONS
  Yeast, Viruses, Bacteria, Parasites
ENZYME/HCL DEFICIENCIES

Note: **"NK Daily"** contains:
  Se Metalo-digestive enz
  High Nitrogen AA
    combo (Arginine, etc.)
  Arabinogalactan

Encourage all soy
  products, especially
  for blood types A and
  AB

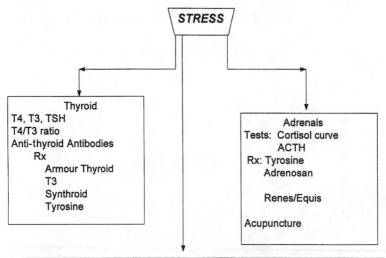

THE
CHALLENGE
to
CHANGE
CHANGE
CHANGE

The capacity to adapt has been exceeded!

STRESS

Thyroid
T4, T3, TSH
T4/T3 ratio
Anti-thyroid Antibodies
Rx
    Armour Thyroid
    T3
    Synthroid
    Tyrosine

Adrenals
Tests: Cortisol curve
        ACTH
Rx: Tyrosine
    Adrenosan

    Renes/Equis

Acupuncture

Issues:
    Existential
        Purpose
        Fulfillment
    Spiritual
    Psychodynamic
        Guilt
        Depression
        Self-Esteem
            Forgiveness
Process oriented psychotherapy
Death and dying issues

Neuroendocrinology
Tyrosine (Catecholamine metabolism)
Serotonin (Melatonin metabolism), 5-HT
Glutamine
St. John's Wort
Mg, P-5-P

Meditation
Visualization
Prayer

The Prostate Gland and Its Other Potential Problems

A Lesson in Anatomy

Both the prostate's functions and its vulnerabilities arise from its place in male anatomy. The prostate is a walnut-sized chestnut-shaped gland, which is strategically located at the point at which the bladder gives rise to the urethra, the outlet for urine. Figure 5 shows the prostate as it lies below the bladder and surrounds the urethra. The urethra is easily recognized as the tube that exits via the penis and allows urination. Figure 6 shows a second tubule (the *vas deferens*, one of the two *ductus deferens*) that leads from the testes, around the bladder, and into the prostate.

The more usual and unglamorous role of the prostate is to control the outflow of urine from the bladder and into the urethra. Urination requires that the prostate's fibromuscular tissue, about 30 percent of its total tissue mass, contract to open (that is, to dilate) the urethral tubing as it passes through the gland. The contraction of the prostate allows fluid to pass through the urethra and, ultimately, through the penis to the outside. (The rest of the urethral structure, which is lined with smooth muscle, remains normally contracted to act as a sphincter and must *relax* to allow the flow of urine.) This role is more properly that of an organ than that of a gland.

As a gland, the prostate is capable of secreting a milky, mildly al-

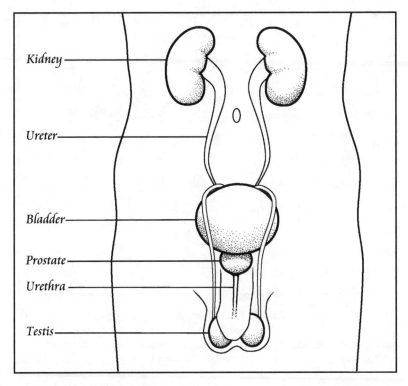

Figure 5. A View of the Prostate. This portrayal of the prostate shows its relationship to other organs.

kaline fluid with some special functions that involve the sperm. As they mature, sperm from the testes flow up the muscle-walled vas deferens, around the bladder and into the *seminal vesicles*, where they are stored. The seminal vesicles produce their own *seminal fluid* that nourishes the sperm and gives volume to the ejaculate. During sexual excitement the seminal vesicles empty their contents into the prostate, which, in turn, adds its own *prostatic fluid* to this mixture. Some prostatic fluid precedes ejaculation, but most of the released fluid is added to the sperm and seminal fluid to constitute the semen. Only about 5 percent of the final ejaculate mixture is composed of actual sperm. Prostatic fluid is both a lubricant and a carrier of sperm and constitutes about 20 percent of the volume of the semen. The muscles of the prostate are very active in the expul-

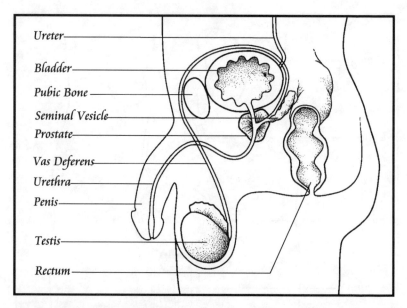

Figure 6. The Prostate and the GI-Tract. In this drawing it is easy to see that the prostate is located very close to the wall of the large intestine. During a biopsy, the collection instrument is brought in through the rectum and the prostate samples are collected directly through the wall of the lower intestine as described in the text.

sion of semen from the body at sexual climax. The stimulation of the prostate, which activates ejaculation, is responsible for much of the intense pleasure that immediately precedes ejaculation.

In an adult male, the prostate usually weighs about 20 grams. Almost all of this mass develops during puberty in response to hormonal changes associated with maturation. The prostate literally doubles in size during puberty. If a man is lucky, and some are, the prostate never again undergoes any changes in size. Unfortunately, of men between the ages of 40 and 59, nearly 60 percent can be shown to already be suffering from the condition known as *benign prostatic hyperplasia* (BPH). This condition usually does not present a noticeable problem until after the age of 50; by the age of 80, however, some 85 percent of all men suffer from one or more symptoms of BPH. As a quick comparison, recall that in the United States *clinically inactive* prostate cancer is found in about 40 percent of men older than 50 years of age and in 70 percent of men who are 80 years old or above. By age 90 the rate approaches 100 percent.

When doctors describe the prostate, they often speak of its *lobes*, by which they simply mean the right and left sides. As the prostate is viewed from the perspective of the bladder, the part that is furthest away is called the *apex*. The portion closest to the bladder is slightly wider and is accordingly called the *base*. Again, the front of the prostate is its *anterior* part, whereas the back is its *posterior* part.

Prostate cancer typically spreads into areas that are closest to this gland/organ and/or receive blood and lymph from it. Figure 7 shows the lymphatic drainage from the prostate, and this association is one reason that cancer of the local lymph nodes is one development from prostate cancer. Other common areas of metastasis are to the pelvic bones and the spine. The reason for the latter is that the blood vessels that return blood from the prostate to the heart run upwards and next

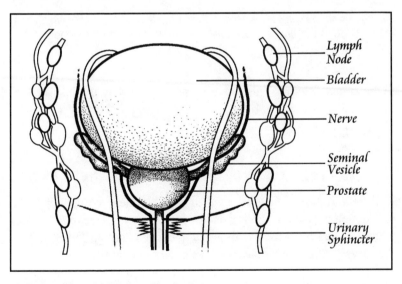

Figure 7. Lymph and Nerve Connections to the Prostate. The prostate plays important roles in sexual functioning. Nerves run along both sides of the prostate and the gland is surrounded by lymph nodes, as well. If the prostate is removed surgically, the nerves must be preserved to allow sexual functioning to be regained. Damage to these nerves can cause not only impotence, but also pain.

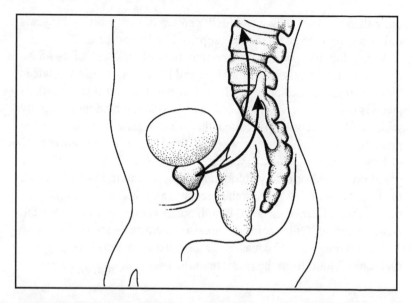

Figure 8. Common Routes of Metastasis. Cells from a prostate cancer which has grown beyond the prostate capsule often metastasize to the bones of the pelvis and to the lower part of the spinal column.

to the spinal column. This aspect of pelvic anatomy is illustrated in Figure 8.

Benign Prostatic Hyperplasia (BPH) Is Not Cancer

BPH and prostate cancer tend to be a "hidden" epidemic. Both can develop without giving any symptoms whatsoever. Just as many or even most men with prostate cancer may go to the end of their lives without ever having developed noticeable symptoms, so, too, men can live with enormously enlarged prostates without any symptoms. In the former case, this is because the cancer typically grows so slowly. In the latter case, it is because only a small section of the prostate impinges upon the urethra and therefore may impede voiding. For these and other reasons, there is a tendency to confuse these two conditions and to fear that BPH may lead to prostate cancer. Yet not only is BPH not cancer, there is no evidence that it leads to cancer.

More than one author has observed that in BPH, the disease is really the symptoms. Benign prostatic hyperplasia (formerly called hypertrophy) in some ways is the male equivalent of menopause. The primary effect of BPH is a progressive decrease in the ability to empty the bladder as the prostate enlarges and applies pressure to the urethra. Retained urine from this obstruction at first can interfere with sleep as the sufferer wakes up in the middle of the night to pee. At other times, pressure may make it impossible to properly control

---

THE AMERICAN UROLOGICAL ASSOCIATION SYMPTOM INDEX

For questions 1–6, score 0 for not at all; 1 for less than 1 time in 5; 2 for less than half the time; 3 for about half the time; 4 for more than half the time; and 5 for almost always.

Your Score

___ 1. Over the past month or so, how often have you had a sensation of not emptying your bladder completely after you finished urinating?

___ 2. Over the past month or so, how often have you had to urinate again less than two hours after you finished urinating?

___ 3. Over the past month or so, how often have you found you stopped and started again several times when you urinated?

___ 4. Over the past month or so, how often have you found it difficult to postpone urination?

___ 5. Over the past month or so, how often have you had a weak urinary stream?

___ 6. Over the past month or so, how often have you had to push or strain to begin urination?

___ 7. Over the last month, how many times did you most typically get up to urinate from the time you went to bed at night until the time you got up in the morning?
(0,1,2,3,4 or 5)

Scoring

The sum of the answer scores gives us the severity of the BPH as follows:

0–7	=	mild prostatism
8–18	=	moderate prostatism
19–35	=	severe prostatism

urine flow (incontinence). Retained urine in the bladder can allow bacterial growth and infection. Urine may flow back up the tubules to the kidneys and cause infection there too. In severe cases of retention and kidney failure, urine even can find its way into the blood (uremia) with toxic consequences. The American Urological Association Symptom Index (reproduced here) is now a standard assessment for BPH severity. Fortunately, BPH prostate problems tend to worsen rather slowly, and this allows a window for applying herbal and nutritional measures. However, severe prostatitis, the inflammation of the prostate, warrants medical consultation.

Nonhormonal/Noncancerous Sources of Prostate Discomfort, Dysfunction and Enlargement

Prostate cancer is hardly the only thing that can go wrong with the prostate. Moreover, not all sources of prostate enlargement arise from hormonal alterations typical of aging, nor are all non-cancerous sources benign. Painful or chronic problems involving urine flow or the urogenital area require the help of a physician. To add insult to injury, a man can have prostate cancer *and* one or more other conditions at the same time.

The first of these conditions is really a catchall that goes under the general name of *prostatitis*. This is an inflammation of the prostate and may involve considerable pain, whereas BPH may not involve any pain at all (as opposed to discomfort). Prostatitis is fairly common in adult males and has been classified into four types. Only at most 5 percent of all cases consist of either *acute* or *chronic bacterial prostatitis*. *Nonbacterial prostatitis* comprises 64 percent of cases and *prostatodynia* makes up another 31 percent.

Acute prostatitis is the result of bacterial infection, usually *E. coli*, and typically begins with the fever, chills and other symptoms that bacterial infections bring on. Pain in the lower back and in the area between the scrotum and the anus are typical, as is difficult and/or painful urination, increased frequency of urination, etc. Acute prostatitis is most commonly found in young sexually active men, and this may be the source of infection, especially if there are many different sexual partners. Treatment includes antibiotics and is usually effective.

Chronic prostatitis can be related to failed treatment of acute prostatitis or it may develop on its own. It involves frequently recurrent low-level infections of the prostate that usually involve the same strain of bacteria. Symptoms include frequent and painful urination and nocturia (waking several times during the night to urinate). Stones or calculi made up of urinary components often are found in the prostatic ducts, and this implies a reflux of urine into these areas. Antibiotics fail as a treatment in cases of chronic prostatitis because they cannot eliminate the bacteria that are found in these stones, hence there is present a constant source for reinfection. Another factor often found is a lack of zinc in prostatic fluid. Prostatic fluid is continuously released and contains a potent antibacterial factor that includes free zinc as the most active ingredient. Men with low levels of zinc in their prostatic fluid seem especially prone to chronic prostatitis.

Nonbacterial prostatitis is the most common of the prostatic conditions, but its cause has not been isolated. It is characterized by an unusually high number and activity of inflammatory cells in the prostate. The resulting inflammation resembles that found in chronic prostatitis, but there is neither a history of infection nor do cultures (for bacteria) prove positive. Along with the symptoms found in bacterial infections, post-ejaculatory pain and discomfort are typical of this form of prostatitis. Conventional medical treatments do not yield good results. Abstaining from alcohol and spicy foods helps in some cases.

Prostatodynia, which is most common in young and middle aged men, presents many symptoms similar to the above, but lacks the excessive number of inflammatory cells. Just as nonbacterial prostatitis has some symptoms that are peculiar to it, so, too, does prostatodynia. In particular, pain and/or discomfort in the groin, perineum, testicles, lower back and penis seem to characterize this condition. Smooth muscle spasms in the prostatic portion of the urethra and in the neck of the bladder are at work here. The subsequent reflux of urine into prostatic and ejaculatory ducts causes a chemically-induced inflammation. Fatigue in the muscles in the pelvic region and emotional stress appear to be powerful contributory factors in prostatodynia.

Hormones and the Prostate

There is a striking overlap in many of the postulated links made between male hormones and prostate cancer and those made for BPH. Therefore it is of considerable importance that many previously accepted arguments regarding the causes of BPH are now undergoing increasing scrutiny and doubt. For decades, it has been accepted medical dogma that prostate cancer is caused by the male hormones testosterone and dihydrotestosterone (DHT). However, drugs that strongly block the production of DHT have not proven to be of much use against either condition. It is much easier to grasp what is at stake if we first look at the less emotionally charged area of non-cancerous prostate enlargement.

Prostate enlargement is strongly related to normal aging. Some of the factors involved are quite well understood. Nevertheless, there also is substantial disagreement about other issues. BPH can be called an aspect of male menopause because an increased ratio of estrogen to testosterone is active in BPH just as, conversely, in women passing through menopause the ratio of testosterone to estrogen increases. It is generally accepted that hormone ratios and hormone clearance are involved in BPH, but the exact ways in which these lead to the enlargement has yet to be definitively explained. As can be seen in Figure 9, testosterone secretion is highly regulated by way of feedback loops involving the pituitary gland and the hypothalamus. Inasmuch as renewed prostate growth appears in later life at the point at which actual testosterone production is in significant decline, it is plausible to suspect that secretory signals may play a role in altering the clearance of testosterone from the tissues affected.

Testosterone, the "male" hormone, is at its peak during adolescence. It decreases thereafter, and the rate of decrease sharpens by about age 50, the point at which most forms of prostate dysfunction begin to become significant. The decline in testosterone production typically calls into play the compensatory release of other hormones

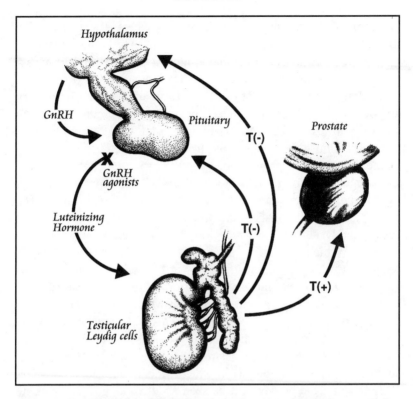

Figure 9. The Regulation of Androgen Production. This figure illustrates the hypothalamic-pituitary-gonadal axis. It includes the site of action (X) of gonadrotropin-releasing hormone (GnRH) agonists and the sites of the inhibitory (-) and the stimulatory (+) actions of testosterone (T). These marked sites are the usual targets of drug intervention.

that are stimulants to testosterone production. These cannot prevent the decline in testosterone levels, but they can lead to an elevated rate of transformation of testosterone into 5-*alpha*-dihydrotestosterone (DHT) and/or to the increased binding and/or to the decreased clearance of DHT from prostate cells. Testosterone is converted to DHT by the enzyme 5-*alpha*-reductase. Ultimately, it is DHT's actions that have been supposed to cause the enlargement of the prostate, just DHT is usually considered to be a primary factor in the development of prostate cancer. DHT binds to specific receptors on the prostate cells usually referred to as *androgen receptors*. It then is transported into the nucleus of these cells where it attaches to the DNA and ultimately turns on prostate growth. As will be explored in more detail below, current research indicates that DHT is a necessary, but not a sufficient cause in the development of BPH.

Increases in the levels of estrogens (primarily estradiol) are very important in these developments. Special enzymes reduce the binding of both testosterone and DHT to prostate cell receptors under normal circumstances, especially in younger men. The unbound androgenic hormones (that is, not bound to prostate cells) can be excreted more readily from the system than the bound forms. Recently, authors have begun to argue that in BPH the rate of removal of DHT in particular is diminished and it is this failure to remove testosterone and DHT from their receptors, and not merely the production of DHT, which primarily encourages the development of BPH. Singularly, estrogen inhibits the actions of the enzymes that metabolize these androgens into excretable forms. In animal models, the combination is a more potent prostate growth stimulant (not here referring to cancer, but to hyperplasia) than are androgens alone. Remember also the observation in the previous chapter that the combination of estrogen and testosterone experimentally produces prostate cancer in animal models in which testosterone alone does not.

In a sense, the body might be seen as attempting to compensate for the decrease in its ability to produce testosterone by increasing the actions of the smaller quantity of the hormone that actually is produced. As is true of the parallel actions of women's bodies during menopause, the secondary modulation of hormonal actions and not the decline in testosterone production *per se* is the cause of BPH and related symptoms. Whether this is true of prostate cancer, as well, is only now becoming a topic of active research.

Another hormone that plays a significant role in the development of BPH is prolactin. Prolactin both increases the conversion of testosterone to DHT and the binding of androgens to prostate cells. Prolactin production itself is increased by stress, alcohol and aging. One counterweight to prolactin is the hormone melatonin, much in the news as an "anti-aging" hormone. Significantly, melatonin, which acts to check prolactin production, declines even as prolactin levels increase with age. This is not to suggest that melatonin supplementation is an answer to BPH or to prostate cancer, but rather to indicate that various factors related to the binding of estrogen to receptors in the prostate increase in later life and must be considered.

It should be kept in mind that many of the factors found in the various forms of prostatitis may come into play in prostate cancer and in BPH. Inflammation is a common and significant element in both conditions. Also of importance are spasms in the smooth muscles that line the urethra and the neck of the bladder, the inability to relax the sphincters constructed of these smooth muscles, a weakened ability to contract the bladder upon command, and so forth. None of these factors are readily influenced by drug approaches to BPH which are intended specifically to inhibit the conversion of testosterone to DHT. In prostate cancer therapy, drugs that block *all* androgens will often radically improve the ability to void, but this actually confirms the connection between estrogens and androgens in the development and continuation of prostate dysfunctions.

A Closer Look at Hormonal and Nonhormonal Factors in BPH

Although the conversion of testosterone to DHT plays an indisputable a role in the development of BPH, the inhibition of this conversion in the treatment of BPH in pharmaceutical trials with the extremely powerful DHT inhibitor *finasteride* (Proscar™) has proven to be far less successful than was expected except in the cases of patients with severely enlarged prostates. Moreover, a number of studies have demonstrated that non-testosterone-based substances secreted by the testes stimulate the growth of prostatic tissues. Hence, although it is clearly the case that men who are severely deficient in androgens (such as through castration or from other causes) do not develop BPH, the actual role of testosterone, DHT, and related factors in the development of BPH in normal males is problematic. Numerous animal experiments have demonstrated the presence of factors other than androgens as being active in prostatic hyperplasia.

Until recently the main target sites for therapeutic intervention in

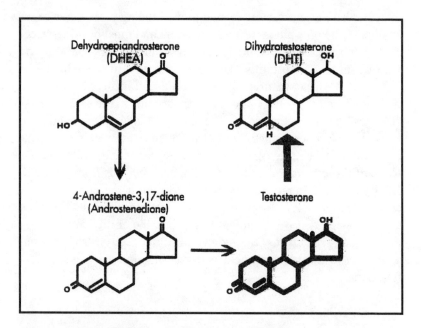

Figure 10. The Synthesis of Dihydrotestosterone (DHT). One line of thought holds that it is DHT in particular which is especially active in both prostate enlargement and prostate cancer. This figure shows the pathway by which DHEA, which is produced primarily in the adrenal glands, is changed into testosterone and then into DHT. These later steps take place primarily in the testes.

cases of BPH have been the actions of 5-a-reductase leading to the production of DHT and/or the DHT/androgen receptor. (DHT accounts for approximately 95 percent of the androgens found in the prostate. See Figure 10.) The role of estrogens has not usually been closely considered. Some authors maintain that the levels of estrogens typically remain largely stable as men age even as testosterone levels fall; other authors find that estradiol levels actually are elevated in men with low testosterone measurements. The emphasis upon blocking DHT, of course, parallels one common approach to treating prostate cancer.

The aromatization of dehydroepiandrosterone (DHEA) and androstenedione is a major source of estrogen in males, although it should not be forgotten that the amount of fatty tissues in the body also can have an impact upon circulating estrogen levels. (Fatty tissues release estrogens, perhaps one reason that obesity is positively linked to the development of prostate cancer.) The ratio of testosterone-to-estrogen, as is true of circulating steroid levels in general, is always closely regulated by the body. Changes in the ratio and in the total levels bring into action counterbalancing mechanisms.

For instance, the liver is stimulated by the changes in the testosterone-to-estrogen ratio via the related elevation 17-estradiol levels. The result is an increase in the production of sex hormone binding globulin (SHBG). Inasmuch as free testosterone has a greater affinity for SHBG than does free estradiol, the net result of this is yet a further decrease in free testosterone levels relative to estrogen levels. Moreover, aromatase enzymes are particularly active in the tissues of the prostate that directly surround the urethra. Low testosterone levels, enhanced estrogen levels, and perhaps the increased presence of SHBG itself, appear to upregulate the androgen receptors in the prostate. Furthermore, estrogen may inhibit the hydroxylation of DHT within the prostate, thus reducing the rate of elimination of this androgen. Animal studies have shown that giving estrogen together with androgens increases prostate growth relative to that caused by giving androgens alone.

Hence, it is now considered to be the case that the elevated ratio of estrogen to testosterone found in aging males increases the activity of androgen receptors in the prostate. Interestingly, estrogens may directly stimulate the growth of smooth muscle cells both within the prostate and the urethra. Spasms and excessive tonus in the smooth muscle of the urethra and the neck of the bladder account for many of the urinary difficulties typically found in cases of BPH, and therefore this growth effect is of considerable significance. Difficulties in voiding often reflect an inability to relax the internal and external sphincters of the prostate and bladder. A recent *in vitro* test with isolated smooth muscle cells from the prostate showed that whereas DHT stimulates the growth of these cells under laboratory conditions, estradiol, an estrogen, is a much more powerful stimulus.

As indicated previously, prolactin is another hormone that influences the production and the binding of DHT. The exact extent of this influence has not been established. Similarly, progesterone may play a role in BPH, perhaps one similar to that of estrogens inasmuch as the contents of the progesterone cytosolic and nuclear receptors are linked to those of the estrogen receptors. Since there are cytosolic and nuclear receptors for androgens, estrogens and progesterone in prostate cells, direct mechanisms of action are available. These are areas of active research.

Evaluating Nonhormonal Factors in BPH and Prostate Cancer

Two sets of non-steroidal elements should be considered as significant factors in both BPH and prostate cancer. The first area is of non-androgenic growth factors. The second is that of inflammation and altered immune response. To these factors should be added alterations in the tonus of the smooth muscles of the prostate, the urethra, etc.

It was long ago suggested that non-androgenic hormones released by the adrenal glands, the hypothalamus and the pituitary may influence the growth of the prostate, including both hyperplasia and the development of precancerous lesions. As is true of prolactin, the levels of luteinizing hormone (LH), follicle-stimulating hormone (FSH) and estrogens (in absolute as well as relative terms) increase in males with age.

Recent research has identified various proteins and growth factors, some originating in the testes, as influencing or even initiating the growth of the prostate that characterizes BPH. Several lines of evidence now indicate that the actions of DHT are at least partially mediated through the mechanisms of these growth factors in the development of BPH. A clinical drug trial published in 1996 that compared saw palmetto (which at clinical dosages has no effect upon blood DHT levels) and finasteride (which is highly significant as an inhibitor of 5-*alpha*-reductase activity) concluded that "BPH, which is an age-related disease, is triggered by non-androgenic factors."

The reader at this point might well wonder whether insulin-like growth factor-1 (IGF-1) mentioned earlier is one of these growth factors. IGF-1 blood levels are strongly related to the development of cancers in general and are known to be elevated at least seven years in advance of the ability to detect prostate cancer by the PSA test. This small protein is a powerful regulator of cell division—and it is not a hormone.

The prostate contains both epithelial and stromal cells. Renewed prostate growth after puberty may involve one or more of the following: epithelium-derived growth factor (EGF, also called epidermal growth factor), insulin-like growth factors-I and -II (IGF-I, IGF-II), basic fibroblast growth factor (bFGF), and keroatinocyte growth factor (KGF). The emerging view of BPH is that tissue proliferation within the prostate may require the presence of androgens, but androgens may not be primarily responsible for the resumed growth of the prostate tissues. This would help to explain the disappointing results found with finasteride (Proscar™) mentioned above. Furthermore, these growth-promoting factors are always balanced by factors that restrain growth, including those that induce programmed cell death. Transforming growth factor (TGF) is one such compound, and significance must be attached to metabolic and hormonal changes that antagonize the normal growth inhibitory factors found in the prostate. *Indeed, programmed cell death may be a natural regulatory mechanism to maintain prostate homeostasis. Programmed cell death, of course, is what is lost in cancer cells.*

Both prostate cancer and BPH in some cases may be the results of long-term inflammatory and immune or autoimmune actions. Constant inflammation is a well recognized initiator of cancerous changes in many tissues. Moreover, theories, which consider free radicals to be possible causes of cancer, fit very well with the view that chronic inflammation is a cause. Excessive immune action creates free radicals and inflammation; inflammation itself activates immune responses.

In the case of BPH, two primary lines of argument have been presented in support of inflammation as causative. First, the prostate may be subject to invasion by bacteria and perhaps viruses, as mentioned previously. Immune cells would follow such agents into prostatic tissues in an attempt to eradicate them, and tissue irritation is typical of sites of active immune intervention. However, pathogens can evade complete eradication by the immune system because the contents of the tubules of the prostate lie outside the normal circulation. Stones formed by the deposition of mineral salts and uric acid crystals, for instance, can harbor bacteria that would lie beyond the reach of the immune system. The low zinc status of most men who suffer from BPH abets chronic low-level infection because free zinc is the most active antibacterial agent found in prostatic fluids.

The other line of argument is that the prostate can become the site of an autoimmune response. The migration of immune cells into the prostate and their constant activity may lead to the deposition of excessive amount of collagen, etc. Again, chronic irritation can be seen as an inducer of prostate cell proliferation.

Both of these lines of argument may have relevance for the development and continuation of prostate cancer.

For the Physician: Protocol/Supplements/Tests

The treatment of prostate cancer is not a self-help subject, but rather requires the care and attention of a compassionate complementary physician.

Each patient must be approached and assessed as an individual, and treated accordingly in order to achieve consistently good results. Part of that assessment process involves specific laboratory tests to clearly understand the patient's present state—both biochemically and immunologically. Effective therapy can then logically follow.

Sometimes pharmaceuticals (drugs) must be used along with natural supplements to buy time for the immune system to recover and engage in battle.

The special lab tests and pharmaceutical weapons below have helped many of my patients through the therapeutic process.

For further information, visit my website at: immune-consultants.com.

Chapter 4—The Promise of PC SPES

PC SPES: 2 tablets, 3 times per day, taken between meals may be best. Available from: 1-800-765-7842.

Matol Omega 3-6-9 Flax Seed Oil combination: 1 tablespoon 2 times per day in veggie juice or over vegetables.

P-Care: 2 tablets 3 times per day.

Flower pollen extract: 2 tablets, 3 times per day.

Chapter 6—Restoring Immune Power

Alkare™: 2 (500 mg) capsules 3 times per day.
Super Anti-Oxidant Formula™: 2 tablets 3 times per day.

Regular Maintenance Formula™ (a good source of B vitamins): 1 tablet 2 times per day

Liver Formula™: 1 tablet 3 times per day.

Ecogen 851™ (fermented soy extract): 1 bottle 2 times per day.

NK Support™: 1 tablespoon, in vegetable juice or water, 3 times per day.

Available from: 1-800-765-7842.

Km™: 2 tablespoons 2 times per day.

Omega 3-6-9™: 1 tablespoon 2 times per day.

Available from: 1-877-9-IMMUNE.

Supreme cleanse™: follow package directions.

Available from: 1-800-831-7780.

Calcium D-glucarate™: 2 capsules 3 times per day.

Available from: 1-800-869-9705.

For further information about TNF-Beta (Kinetrex™), call 1-520-740-1315.

Hydrazine sulfate: 1 (60 mg) capsule 3 times per day to start. Then increase dose to 2 capsules 3 times per day.

Available from: 1-619-656-1980.

Pulsatilla™: 5 drops 3 times per day.

Available from: 1-800-611-8235.

Sun's Soup, a Chinese herbal "soup" that has been shown to be helpful with cachexia.

Available from: 1-203-882-9672.

From your local health food store:

A high-potency, broad spectrum acidophilus (Jarro-Dophilus) preparation 3 times per day.

FOS (by Nutra Flora™): ¼ teaspoon in vegetable juice or water 3 times per day.

Max-EPA™ fish oil: 2 capsules 3 times per day.

Chapter 7—Boosting the Immune System

NK Cell Support™: 1 tablespoon in veggie juice or water 3 times per day.

Available from: 1-800-765-7842.

Biomune™: 2 capsules taken 3 times per day.
Available from: 1-877-9-IMMUNE.

Choleodoron™: 7 drops by mouth 3 times per day.
Vitis comp™: 1 tablet by mouth 3 times per day.
Available by prescription from: 1-914-268-8572.

Ukrain (see above directions) may be purchased and imported from:
011-43-1-5861224.

Step 1. Breaking Anergy:
    If the patient has blood type O or B: Pneumovax™ 0.05 cc s.c./i.d.
Q.O.D. until there is a local reaction like a bee sting.
    If he has blood type A or AB: BCG™ 0.05 cc s.c./i.d. Q.O.D. until there
is a local reaction like a bee sting.

Step 2.
Go on to strategies that break tolerance and support immune reactivation, as
    briefly and incompletely stated:

    Cytokine protocol, if indicated by severe immune dysfunction with low
B- and NK cells:
        1 MU s.c. Q.O.D. INF-alpha alternating with IL-2
        Tagamet™ 200 mg P.O. B.I.D.
        Indocin™: 25mg P.O. B.I.D.
        Melatonin: 20 mg P.O. H.S.
        Available by prescription from: 1-602-948-7065.

    or

TNF-Beta Kinetrex™.
Information available from: 1-520-740-1315.

    or

Autologous cytokines.
Information available from 770-474-4422 or 1-877-9-IMMUNE.

    and

Lien comp™: 1 amp.
Renes/Equis comp™: 1 amp.
Cardus m./Viscum comp™: 1 amp.
Iscucin M.™ ser. H: 1 amp.
Available by prescription from: 1-916-962-1099.

These are combined and given in 100cc NS over ½–¾ hr Q.D. Give Q.O.D. if the patient is severely compromised (with cachexia) or develops a low-grade fever after the I.V. (which, as a sign of the stimulation of the immune system, is a good thing).

Blood tests to monitor:
ECP
CRP
NK cell function
TNF-a
sIL2-r
sIL6-r
Fractionated PSA
PAP
These tests are available from Tiburon Labs 1-520-884-1094.
CBC
This test is available at labs, hospitals, or doctor's offices.

Contact other labs for assistance per your individual needs, such as liver function tests, etc.

Chapter 8—Hormones: Your "River of Life"

Useful lab tests:
Great Smokies—Liver Detox Panel: 1-800-522-4762.
From your local lab: TSH, FT3, and FT4.

Chapter 9—Cell Death: A Time to Live and a Time to Die

P-Care (a balanced source of vitamins A and D and an excellent source for CoQ 10 and Niacin), 2 tablets 3 times per day.

Super Anti-Oxidant Formula (a good source of Quercetin) 2 tablets 3 times per day.
The above are available from the manufacturer and distributor at: 1-800-765-7842.

Ecogen 851 (a specially fermented soy extract product very high in genistein) 1 bottle twice per day.
Available from Lausam: 1-908-688-7171.

Iscar is available by prescription from the Weleda Pharmacy at: 914-268-8572.
Iscucin is available by prescription from the Raphael Pharmacy at: 916-962-1099.

Physicians' Organizations for Complementary Medicine

Cancer Treatment Centers of America
1-800-FOR-HELP

American Association of Orthomolecular Medicine
415-922-6462

American College of Advancement in Medicine
714-583-7666

International Foundation for Innovative Medicine
908-810-9201

Cancer Control Society
213-663-7801

Foundation for Advancement in Cancer Therapy
212-741-2790

International Academy of Nutrition and Preventive Medicine
704-258-3243

National Center of Homeopathy
703-548-7790

Physicians Association of Anthroposophical Medicine
734-662-9355

Foundation for Alternative Cancer Therapies
212-741-2790

Glossary

abdomen: The part of the body located below the ribs and above the pelvic bone.

acid phosphatase/prostate acid phosphatase (PAP): An enzyme made by both normal and malignant cells in the prostate. Malignant cells that break out of the prostate and move to other places in the body continue to make acid phosphatase, thus elevating its value above the normal level in a blood test. Elevated blood serum levels of acid phosphatase may indicate that prostatic cancer cells have spread outside the prostate gland. PAP cannot be used as a screening test to detect early prostatic cancer still confined within the gland itself.

acute: A disorder or infection in the body that reaches a crisis rapidly rather than through a slow, progressive onset.

acute bacterial prostatitis: A form of prostatitis associated with urinary tract infections, the presence of bacteria in urinary cultures, and an abundance of white blood cells in prostatic secretions. Its onset is sudden rather than by slow growth of prostatic tissue as in BPH.

adenocarcinoma: The most common type of prostate tumor and the type most responsive to hormonal therapy. It develops in glandular tissue (specifically the acinar glands) located in the posterior peripheral zone of the prostate.

adjuvant therapy: A treatment method used in addition to the primary therapy.

adrenal glands: Two glands located above the kidneys (one above each kidney). They produce several kinds of hormones, including a small amount of sex hormones.

age-specific or age-adjusted reference range for PSA: The normal values of PSA modified or correlated to the age of the patient in order to more accurately determine the significance of PSA numbers.

alpha-adrenergic blockers: Medications which relax the smooth muscle tissues of the bladder neck and the prostate to relieve the pressure on the urethral channel and open the passage to increase urine flow.

alternative treatment: Any treatment other than surgery, radiation, and chemotherapy which relies on other healing processes. These include nutrition, exercise, herbs, supplements, etc.

androgens: Include all of the male hormones. These are necessary for the development and functioning of male sexual organs and male characteristics (facial hair, deep voice). The term also is used as a general reference to testosterone and dihydrotestosterone *(see* Testosterone and Dihydrotestosterone).

aneuploid: An aggressive prostate cancer tumor which has either more or less than the normal 46 chromosomes.

angiogenesis: The formation of new blood vessels.

antagonist: In medicine or medical research, an agent that nullifies the action of another agent.

antiandrogens or androgen blockers: Medications that reduce or eliminate the production of androgens. Drugs such as Casodex, Eulexin, and Nilandron are used in hormone therapy to treat prostate cancer by blocking the impact of testosterone and DHT on prostate cancer cells.

antiangiogenesis: Preventing the development of new blood vessels.

Anti-Mailgnin Antibody in Serum (AMAS) test: A blood test which can be used to determine the presence of cancer in the body. However, it is not test which is specific to prostate cancer.

anus: The opening of the rectum through which solid waste leaves the body.

apex of the prostate: The tip of the prostate that is farthest away from the bladder; commonly called the *bottom of the prostate.*

asymptomatic: The absence of symptoms typical of a disorder such as BPH or cancer.

atrophy: A decrease in, or slow wasting away of, body tissue.

base of the prostate: Wide part of the top of the prostate, adjacent to the bladder.

benign: Usually used with regard to a growth or tumor to indicate the absence of cancer, that is, it is nonmalignant and/or nonrecurrent.

benign prostatic hyperplasia (BPH): The nonmalignant abnormal multiplication of cells in the prostate gland. Commonly called *enlargement of the prostate gland,* this condition can result in the gradual compression of the urethra within the prostate. BPH can elevate PSA scores. However, elevated PSA numbers resulting from BPH do not necessarily indicate the presence of cancer, although cancer may be present.

bilateral orchiectomy: Surgical removal of the testicles to halt the production of testosterone.

biopsy: Removal of small samples of tissue for later microscopic examination to establish a precise diagnosis and, more specifically, to determine if cancer is present.

bladder: The muscular sac or hollow organ which collects and stores urine in the body before it is discharged.

bladder neck: Circular muscular fibers which come together like a funnel where the bladder opens into the prostate. Any constriction of the bladder neck can impede urine flow.

bone scan: Several hours after ingestion of a substance which accumulates in abnormal bones, a picture is taken to determine if prostate cancer is present in the bones.

brachytherapy: The insertion of radioactive pellets into the prostate for cancer treatment. Also called *interstitial radiation therapy.*

cancer: A cellular tumor which is normally ultimately fatal. Unlike benign tumor cells, cancer cells are capable of invading and destroying organs and of *metastasizing,*

capsule of the prostate: The fibrous tissue that comprises the outer wall of the prostate gland.

Casodex: A recently FDA-approved antiandrogen used to block the uptake of testosterone at the receptors of the adrenal gland.

castration: Elimination of testicular function, either by surgical removal of the testes (surgical castration), or by administration of a LH-RH analog (a class of drugs designed to inhibit testicular function).

carcinoma: Cancer cells that form in the lining of an organ or cavity.

catheter: A tube inserted into a body cavity, passageway, or organ. Most commonly used for irrigation or drainage after surgery, to empty organs such as the bladder (following surgery or due to constriction), or to keep a canal open.

Caverject: The brand name of the product in which Alprostadil is dispensed.

cell: The smallest unit of the body. All of the cells combined form all the tissues and organs of the body. When cells divide, new tissue is created.

chemotherapy: The use of specific and powerful drugs to attack and destroy cancer cells. Since they can also kill other cells in the body, chemotherapeutic agents are potentially quite dangerous.

chronic: The persistence of an illness or infection over a long period of time.

clinical trial: A planned research study to evaluate a new treatment or medication for an as yet unproven use.

Cobalt 60: A radioactive substance used as a radiation source to treat cancer.

complication: An unwanted, undesirable, often unpleasant, and occasionally permanent result of a treatment, procedure, or medication.

Computerized Tomography/CT scan: A computer-assisted type of X-ray allowing detailed visualization of the body; particularly useful in evaluating organs.

conventional treatment of cancer: A treatment falling into any one of three categories: surgery, radiation, and chemotherapy.

cryo-probes: Probes used in cryosurgery to freeze tissue in the prostate gland.

cryotherapy: Sometimes called *cryosurgery,* this term refers to the use of liquid nitrogen to freeze the prostate by placing probes through the perineum and into the prostate. Cryotherapy is used to eliminate cancer, but in doing so, it kills all the prostate tissue, including both cancer and normal cells.

cystoscope: An instrument composed of a slender hollow tube with a lens at each end to allow direct visual examination of the interior of the urethra and bladder. The examination itself is called a *cystoscopy.*

deferred therapy: Another name for "watchful waiting" or delaying actual treatment but including regular monitoring.

digital rectal exam (DRE): When a doctor inserts a gloved, lubricated finger into the rectum to feel for lumps, enlargement, or areas of hardness that might indicate the presence of cancer in the prostate.

dihydrotestosterone (DHT): The more powerful hormone that results from the active breakdown of testosterone by an enzyme called 5-*alpha*-reductase.

diploid: Slow-growing prostate cancer cells which have the normal 46 chromosomes.

DNA (deoxyribonucleic acid): The basic biologically active chemical which defines the physical development and growth of humans and nearly all other living organisms.

DNA ploidy analysis: A study used to determine the growth characteristics of prostate cancer cells by determining the number of chromosomes.

double-blind research study: Research where neither the doctor nor the patient/subject (and sometimes the evaluator) knows which medication or treatment is being used with any individual patient. Its purpose is to minimize the effects of personal opinion or bias on the results of the study.

epithelium (or epithelial tissue): Membranous cell tissue which covers external and internal surfaces of the body, including the lining of blood vessels and other small cavities. It is classified into several types on the basis of the number of layers of depth and the shape of the cells. Depending on where it is located, its functions include enclosing and protecting, producing secretions and excretions, and assisting in assimilation.

erectile dysfunction: A more specific term for *impotence,* which refers to the inability to have and/or to maintain an erection for sexual intercourse.

estrogen: A female sex hormone. There are many related compounds which are "estrogens" (*see* Phytoestrogens).

external-beam radiation therapy: The use of an external source, called a *linear accelerator,* to aim high-level radiation waves at a cancer.

false negative: When the results of a test are erroneously reported as negative (that is, having no evidence of the condition being tested for) despite the fact that the condition does exist.

false positive: The erroneous report of a test as positive (indicating the condition tested for does exist).

flow cytometry: The process by which graphs or histograms are plotted based on the DNA reading of the cancerous tissue cells.

5-*alpha* reductase: An enzyme in the prostate gland which converts testosterone to DHT (the more active form of male hormone).

flow rate (urine): The measurement of urine as it is expelled from the bladder at its peak period of movement. A rate which is lower than normal suggests that an obstruction might be present.

Foley catheter: A catheter placed in the bladder for continuous drainage, usually after a prostatectomy, which is kept in place by means of a balloon which is inflated with liquid.

genitourinary tract: The combination of the urinary system (kidneys, ureters, bladder, and urethra) and the genital system (including, in the male, testicles, vas deferens, prostate, and penis).

gland: An aggregation or group of specialized cells which secrete materials unnecessary for their own metabolic needs but which influence the development or actions of other cells and organs in the body.

hematospermia: The presence of blood in the semen.

hematuria: The presence of blood in the urine.

hesitancy: When a man has to wait for several seconds or longer for his urine to flow because the bladder is straining against the resistance caused by an enlarged prostate.

hormonally insensitive: Refers to prostate cancer cells which are no longer sensitive to hormonal therapy designed to reduce androgen levels.

hormonally refractory: A condition in which hormonal therapy or medical castration no longer controls the growth of prostate cancer.

hormonally sensitive: Prostate cancer cells which are sensitive to hormonal therapy.

hormones: Biologically active chemicals produced in the body. Hormones circulate in bodily fluids and exercise specific effects upon the activity of other cells or organs remote from the hormone-producing cells.

hormone therapy: Treatment which prevents cancer cells from getting the hormones they need to grow. Hormone therapy for prostate cancer keeps the cancer cells from getting male hormones. Treatment may involve removing the testicles or giving female hormones or other drugs to prevent the production of male hormones or to block their effects upon cancer cells.

hyperplasia: The abnormal enlargement of an organ or tissue because of an increase in the number of its cells.

hyperthermia: Using the heat produced by microwave radiation to treat cancer.

immune system: The human body's natural defenses used to fight disease, bacteria, and viruses.

implant: A small container of radioactive material placed in or near a cancer.

impotence: The partial or complete loss of erection which may be associated with a loss of libido. Impotence may result from injury secondary to radiation therapy or surgical resection of the prostate or may be a result of hormone deprivation therapy.

incision: A cut made during surgery.

incontinence: Partial or complete loss of urine control.

inflammation: Swelling, pain, or irritation as a result of the reaction of tissue to injury or infection. Commonly involves elements of immune response and/or free radical damage.

intermittent hormonal therapy: The process of administering combined hormone therapy (CHT) during intervals instead of on a continuous basis.

internal radiation: A type of therapy in which a radioactive substance is implanted into or close to the area needing treatment.

interstitial: Situated within the spaces or "gaps" in the tissue of a particular organ.

in vitro: Refers to studies on prostate tissue that are conducted outside a living body and in an artificial environment—usually a test tube or a culture dish.

in vivo: Refers to studies on prostate tissue that remains in the living body of a human or animal while studied.

LH-RH agonists: See luteinizing hormone-releasing hormone (LH-RH) agonist.

linear accelerator: A machine which creates high-energy radiation in the form a stream of fast-moving subatomic particles to treat cancers.

local therapy: Treatment which affects a tumor and tissue near it.

luteinizing hormone-releasing hormone (LH-RH): The hormone released by the pituitary which acts on the testes to stimulate testosterone production.

luteinizing hormone-releasing hormone (LH-RH) agonist: A substance which closely resembles LH-RH. However, LH-RH agonists affect the body differently than does LH-RH. LH-RH agonists keep the testicles from producing hormones by at first overstimulating production, an action which subsequently causes the drastic down-regulation of LH-RH.

lymph: A clear fluid which drains waste from cells. Lymph travels through vessels called *lymphatic channels* and drains into small, bean-shaped structures called *lymph nodes.*

lymph nodes: Small masses of tissue or nodules located along the vessels or channels of the lymphatic drainage system. The lymph nodes are common sites for the spread of cancers.

lymphadenectomy: The surgical removal of one or more lymph nodes for purposes of microscopic examination; may be performed as an "open pelvic lymphadenectomy" as the initial approach during radical prostatectomy or a separate procedure prior to radical prostatectomy by means of small incision(s) into the pelvic cavity (laparoscopic lymphadenectomy).

lymphatic system: The tissues and organs which produce, store, and carry cells that fight infection and disease via the lymph. This system includes the bone marrow, spleen, thymus, lymph nodes, and channels that carry lymph.

MRI (magnetic resonance imaging) scan: A sophisticated use of electromagnetic waves to create a detailed X-ray-type image by measurement of signal intensity of a particular body part or region; in general, this may be the most effective means of detection.

malignant: Usually refers to cancerous tissues; opposite of *benign*.

membrane: A thin, pliable layer of tissue which covers a surface, lines a cavity, or divides a space.

metastasis: A secondary tumor formed and growing at a new site. It develops as a result of cancer cells from a first, or primary, site, traveling through the body to a secondary site(s).

moderately differentiated: A classification of prostate cancer in which the cells are beginning to lose their shape. This corresponds to a Gleason score of *5,* 6, or 7.

nanograms per milliliter (ng/ml): A minute quantity of a substance: one one-billionth of a gram (454 grams make a pound) in one one-thousandth of a liter (one liter is about a quart).

nerve-sparing prostatectomy: A refinement of prostatectomies designed in the early 1980s which saves the nerves necessary for a man to achieve penile erection. It is also called *anatomic prostatectomy* to distinguish it from the older style of prostatectomy which does not save the necessary nerve bundles and which still may be necessary if cancer has spread to them.

nocturia: The need to urinate frequently during the night.

oncologist: A physician specifically trained in the diagnosis and treatment of cancer.

orchiectomy: The surgical removal of one or both of the testicles. It is one way to control the development of male hormones in order to slow down the growth of prostate cancer.

palliative: Any treatment with the purpose of relieving symptoms rather than bringing about a cure.

PC SPES: A new, promising alternative therapy that has successfully controlled prostate cancer. It is most effective taken *before* a patient goes on anti-androgen drugs.

peak flow rate (urine): The maximum rate of flow which a person is able to generate as measured in milliliters per second.

Partin Tables: A multitable used to determine the probability that a prostate cancer patient's disease has spread either to the lymph nodes, seminal vesicles, or beyond.

pathologist: A doctor who identifies disease by studying cells and tissues under a microscope.

pelvic: Referring to the area of the body located below the waist and surrounded by the hip and pubic bones.

perineal prostatectomy: Surgery to remove the prostate through an incision made between the scrotum and the anus.

perineum: In a man, that part of the pelvis located between the bottom of the scrotum and the beginning of the anus.

phytoestrogens: Plant-derived estrogens which mimic one or more actions of the human hormones. Often can be used to block the negative effects of xenoestrogens (environmental toxins which are found in pesticides and plastic products).

placebo: Commonly used in research or clinical trials to determine the effectiveness of a drug, it is an inactive delivery form which looks like the active delivery form containing the medication being investigated. For the research to be a success, the active delivery form must be more effective than the placebo.

poorly differentiated: A classification of prostate cancer in which there is no definite shape of the cells. This corresponds to a Gleason score of between 8 and 10.

primary: A term which refers to the organ or gland where the cancer begins and from which it may then spread (for example, "primary" prostate cancer, which may "metastasize" to the bone).

prognosis: The probable outcome or course of a disease; the chance of recovery.

progression: A term used most commonly to describe continued growth of the cancer, or the recurrence of a cancer after a previous response to treatment.

prostaglandin(s): One of several hormone-like fatty acids which in small amounts act on various organs and upon the immune system. They cause a variety of changes in smooth muscle tone, hormonal functions, and in the functioning of the autonomic and central nervous systems. Prostaglandins produced by the prostate are present in seminal fluid. They are thought to encourage the opening of the female uterus (the cervix) to dilate, making it easier for the sperm to pass into the uterus.

prostate: A walnut-shaped muscular gland which only males have. It is composed of muscle, connective tissue, and glandular tissue and surrounds the urethra immediately below the bladder.

The main function of the inch-and-a-half-long gland is to make part of the fluid for semen. It also provides some of the nutrient material in the semen for sperm during their journey out of the body.

prostate-specific antigen (PSA): An enzyme secreted by the prostate gland, some of which passes into the bloodstream. Enlargement of the gland (BPH), prostatitis, and other conditions, especially cancer, can raise the PSA level detected in the blood.

prostatitis: An infection of the prostate gland usually caused by the presence of bacteria. The presence of this infection can raise the numbers of a PSA test.

prostatostasis: A common form of nonbacterial prostatitis; it is generally attributed to the accumulation of excess fluid or, more specifically, to the engorgement of the prostate's fluid-producing glands due to irregular or infrequent ejaculation.

PSA density: The ratio of PSA to the volume of the prostate gland.

PSA II: The blood test used to determine if a patient has benign prostatic hyperplasia by measuring the amount of free PSA.

PSA doubling time: The process of determining the rate of progression of prostate cancer by measuring the doubling time of the increase in PSA scores.

PSA transitional zone: A method of determining prostate cancer by deciding the value of the transition zone of the prostate gland by the PSA level.

PSA velocity: The degree of change in the PSA level from year to year.

rad: Short for "radiation absorbed dose"; a measurement of the amount of radiation absorbed by tissues (100 rad = 1 gray).

radiation: Energy carried by waves or a stream of particles.

radiation therapy: Treatment with high-energy rays from X rays or other sources to damage cancer cells. The radiation may be from a machine (external radiation therapy) or from radioactive materials placed inside the body as close as possible to the cancer (internal radiation therapy).

radical prostatectomy: The complete surgical removal of the prostate gland, usually done to prevent the spread of prostate cancer.

rectum: The last few inches of the intestine leading to the anus, from which waste solids leave the body.

recurrence: Reappearance of a cancer after the failure of an initial treatment protocol.

refractory: A term used most commonly to describe the situation in which the disease is no longer controlled by current therapy.

remission: Disappearance of the signs and symptoms of cancer. When this happens, the disease is said to be "in remission."

residual urine: Any urine remaining in the bladder immediately after urination.

retropubic: A surgical procedure in which the surgeon makes an incision in the lower abdomen.

retropubic prostatectomy: Surgical removal of the prostate through an incision in the abdomen.

RT-PCR PSA blood test: A test used to determine if a patient's prostate cancer is in the bloodstream; this would indicate that the disease has spread outside the prostate capsule.

salvage therapy: A treatment used to eradicate residual prostate cancer.

scrotum: The saclike structure which contains a man's testes or testicles.

seed implantation: A treatment for prostate cancer in which radioactive seeds are inserted in the prostate gland to kill malignant cells.

semen: The fluid released through the penis during orgasm. Semen is made up of sperm from the testicles and fluid from the prostate and other sex glands.

sextant biopsy: An attempt to get a comprehensive picture of the prostate by extracting six tiny samples of cells through the gland.

simulation: A process involving special X ray pictures which are used to plan radiation treatment so that the areas to be treated are precisely located and marked.

spectroscopic MRI: The combination of high-resolution anatomic (MRI) and metabolic (MRSI) imaging to improve the accuracy of staging in prostate cancer patients.

spot radiation: Radiation aimed at a specific spot on the human body.

staging: The process of determining the size and extent (or stage) of prostate cancer.

stroma: In anatomy, a general term for the tissue which forms the structural elements of an organ. It is the tissue which forms the framework or matrix of an organ, as distinguished from the tissue which constitutes its functional element. In the prostate, stroma is sometimes called *smooth muscle tissue* to distinguish it from the epithelial or glandular tissue.

surgical capsule: The term is used to indicate the point at which expanding new growth of the prostate in BPH meets normal and true prostate tissue.

testes: A man's reproductive organs. Located inside the scrotum, the testes are divided into hundreds of minuscule compartments and are the main source of testosterone and of sperm.

testosterone: The male hormone, which comprises about 90 percent of the male hormones, or androgens, in a man's body.

tetraploid: An aggressive prostate cancer tumor which has four times the normal number of chromosomes.

total ablation therapy: A form of hormone therapy to treat prostate cancer by combining hormones or surgery to yield whatever will achieve a castration level of testosterone.

total androgen blockade or ablation: A form of hormonal therapy in which the entire production of testosterone is shut down using either surgical castration plus an antiandrogen or chemical castration consisting of an LH-RH agonist plus an antiandrogen.

toxic: Refers to a poisonous substance.

transrectal ultrasound (TRUS): Test which uses a probe inserted in the rectum to produce high-frequency sound waves too high for the human ear to hear. These sound waves are then converted into a picture of the prostate gland and surrounding tissue.

transurethral: The route through the urethra.

transurethral incision of the prostate (TUIP): A procedure involving making two incisions from the bladder neck through the prostate in order to widen the urinary passage and decrease the symptoms of BPH.

transurethral resection: Removing BPH tissue obstructing the urethra via instruments inserted into the urethra.

transurethral resection of the prostate (TURP): A procedure for BPH wherein the surgeon tunnels through the urethra into the prostate to cut away enlarged tissue.

urethra: A membranous canal about eight inches long which transports urine from the bladder to the exterior of the body. In men, it extends from the base of the bladder through the prostate gland (where it's called the *prostatic urethra)* into the center of the penis *(penile urethra)* and to the opening at its tip.

urologist: A doctor specializing in diseases of the urinary organs in females and the urinary and sex organs in males.

watchful waiting: *See* "Deferred therapy."

well-differentiated: A classification of prostate cancer in which the cells have definite shape and corresponds to a Gleason score of between 2 and 4.

X-ray: High-energy radiation which can be used at low levels to diagnose disease or at high levels to treat cancer.

zones of the prostate gland: There are five zones of the prostate gland. The peripheral zone is most commonly affected by prostate cancer.

RESOURCE SECTION

Dr. Stoff's Prescription Resources

TNF-Beta (Kinetrex™) (a cytokine that specifically helps kill cancer cells)
Contact Immune Consultants: 1-520-740-1315

Hydrazine sulfate (to help with cachexia)
Androcure (an anti-hormonal progestational drug)
Both are available from AMARC: 1-619-656-1980

Ukrain (to help immune system targeting)
May be purchased and imported from Nowicky Pharmaceuticals: 011-43-1-5861224

Choleodoron™ and Vitis comp™ (to help liver detoxification)
Contact Weleda Pharmacy: 1-914-268-8572

Pneumovax and BCG
(to help break anergy—the failure of the body to respond to an antigen)
Contact your local pharmacy or Mountainview Pharmacy: 1-480-948-7065

B-1.3-Glucan (stimulates macrophage function)
Contact Mountainview Pharmacy: 1-480-948-7065

Cytokine (Immune Stimulating) Protocol
(for supporting and directing a damaged immune system in its fight against cancer)
These are available by prescription from your local pharmacy or Mountainview Pharmacy 1-480-948-7065:

INF-alpha, IL-2
Tagamet™
Indocin™ or Celebrex™
Melatonin 20 mg

Autologous vaccine (to rebuild the immune system)
Information from Immune Nutraceuticals: 1-877-9-IMMUNE

Homeopathic Medicines:

Lien comp™ (to support spleen function)*
Renes/Equis comp™ (to support kidney function)*
Cardus m./Viscum™ (for liver detoxification)*

Isucin M. ™ ser.H (Mistletoe extract)
(stimulates Natural Killer cells)
All of the above homeopathic medicines are available from Raphael Pharmacy: 1-916-962-1099

Iscar (Mistletoe) (stimulates Natural Killer Cells)
Available by prescription from Weleda Pharmacy: 1-914-268-8572

Proscar™, Flutamine™, and Zoladex™
(for combined hormonal blockade)
Available from any local pharmacy

Zovirax™ and Gancyclovir™ (antiviral drugs)
Available from any local pharmacy

(*These homeopathic medicines are best used with constitutional acupuncture)

Dr. Stoff's Laboratory Resources

The following laboratories offer these frequently required tests:

Immune Consultants: 1-520-740-1315
NK cell function

Tiburon Diagnostic Laboratory:
1-520-884-1094
ECP
TNF-a
sIL2-r
sIL6-r
Fractionated PSA
Stoff's Special T&B Cell subset panel
Alpha-Interferon

ImmunoScience Laboratory: 1-310-657-1077
G.I. Evaluation

Great Smokies Diagnostic Laboratory: 1-800-522-4762

Comprehensive Digestive Stool Analysis
Liver Detox Panel

Metametrix Labs: 1-800-221-4640
Urine Organic acids

From your local lab, physicians office or hospital:
TSH, FT3 and FT4
CBC
Full Chemistry Panel
Blood type
CRP
PAP

Treatment Center for Radiation
Cancer Treatment Centers of America:
1-800-367-4357

Some Important New Products Not Previously Mentioned in This Book

PROGESTERONE CREAM

Dr. Stoff recommends this product for users of PC SPES who experience side effects of swelling or tenderness of their breasts. Available from the following companies:

N.E.E.D.S.
1-800-634-1380
www.needs.com

Transitions For Health, Inc.
1-800-455-5182
www.emerita.com
Emerita®
Progest® Body Cream
Contains aloe vera gel, d-alpha tocopherol and mixed tocopherols, almond oil, panthenol, USP progesterone, oil of lemon, keratin, grapefruit seed extract, and other natural ingredients.

Matol
1-800-363-1890
www.matol.com
Botanelle™ Progesterone Crème
A unique infusion of aloe vera, MSM (methylsulfonylmethane) and synergistic botanical extracts; chasteberry, fenugreek, red clover, Siberian ginseng, and wild yam. Other natural ingredients include rosemary oil, jojoba oil, grapefruit seed extract and vitamin E.

PROTEIN SUPPLEMENT
Proper Nutrition, Inc.
1-800-555-8868
www.propernutrition.com
Seacure®
This is an unusual protein supplement made from white fish that has been recommended by M.D.'s such as Julian Whitaker, Christine Northrup and Sherry Rogers. It is also highly recommended for cancer patients by Dr. Patrick Quillin,

the author of the foreword of this book. Seacure® is ideal for cancer patients who often experience problems with digestion and absorption, because it is a pre-digested source of peptides and amino acids that are completely absorbed and utilized by the body. Seacure® is available in 500 mg capsules.

Ribose™

Bioenergy, Inc.
1-888-237-6963
www.ribose.com
This is a 5-carbon carbohydrate that is very effective in boosting energy levels. Available in powder form. Take a rounded teaspoon with juice or water. Contact Bioenergy, Inc. for a list of companies that market this product.

Resources

The following companies have a number of products listed in this resource section. Companies with only one product listed have their toll-free numbers and websites listed along with their products.

The Apothecary
Nutritional Pharmacists
1-800-869-9159
www.The-apothecary.com

Carlson® Laboratories
1-800-323-4141
www.carlsonlabs.com

EcoNugenics®
1-800-308-5518
www.econugenics.com

Gaia Herbs, Inc.
1-800-831-7780
www.gaiaherbs.com

Jarrow Formulas™
1-800-726-0886
www.jarrow.com

Matol
1-800-363-1890
www.matol.com

MegaFood
1-800-848-2542
www.megafood.com

Natural Balance, Inc.
1-800-833-8737
www.naturalbalance.com

N.E.E.D.S.
1-800-634-1380
www.needs.com

Prevail Corporation
1-800-248-0885
www.prevail.com

Solstice
1-800-765-7842
www.solsticevitamin.com

Source Naturals®
1-800-815-2333
www.sourcenaturals.com

The Synergy Company™
1-800-723-0277
www.synergy-co.com

Tree of Life®
www.treeoflife.com

Tyler, Inc.
1-800-869-9705
www.tyler-inc.com

Wakunaga of America, Inc.
1-800-421-2998
www.kyolic.com

Resources: Supplements

Listed here are nutritional supplements used by Lee Heiman (whose case history appears in this book), most of which are recommended by Dr. Jesse Stoff. We have endeavored to find the best companies that carry these supplements. If you cannot find a particular product at your local healthfood store, please contact the company directly for the names of stores or mail order companies that carry it.

ADAPTOGENS

To help shield the body against stress. The ones listed below act synergistically in liver cleansing and are great antioxidants:

Swedish Herbal Institute
1-800-774-9444
www.adaptogen.com
Arctic Root®
Available in tablet form.
Chisandra Adaptogen®
Available in tablet form.

AIDBCWE—ALSO KNOWN AS Ai/E10™

Specifically supports the response of natural killer cells. Available from the following companies:

Body Wise
1-800-830-9596
www.bodywise.com
AG-Immune™
Dietary supplement for a healthy immune system. Two capsules contain 300 mg Immune Enhancer™ AG (arabinogalactan), 100 mg Ai/E10™ (Whey), 50 mg astragalus root, 50 mg maitake mushroom extract 4.1, and other ingredients. This is the only Ai/E10™ formulation that combines these immune-boosting ingredients.

Matol
Biomune OSF™ Plus
A very effective formulation in boosting and enhancing immune function. Each capsule contains 100 mg of dairy colostrum and whey extract (Ai/E10™), 200 mg of astragalus (root), and other ingredients.
Biomune OSF™ Express
Nasal spray. Homeopathic medicine for a healthy immune system. Contains Ai/E10™.

ALLERGY RELIEF

For allergy sufferers who can have reduced immune function.

Carlson® Laboratories
Aler-Key®
Hypoallergenic nutritional support for the allergen sensitive. Two capsules contain 800 mg vitamin C, 300 mg quercetin, 200 mg pantothenic acid, 10 mg vitamin B-2, 10 mg vitamin B-6, and 116 mg calcium.

ALPHA LIPOIC ACID

Available from the following companies:

Jarrow Formulas
Alpha Lipoic Sustain 300
Each tablet contains 300 mg of alpha lipoic acid in a sustained release format to minimize gastric irritations and blood sugar fluctuations.

Source Naturals®
Alpha Lipoic Acid
For immune system support. Stimulates glutathione production. Available in 50 mg, 100 mg and 200 mg tablets.

AMINO ACIDS

Carlson® Laboratories
Amino Blend
Scientifically balanced formulation of 22 essential and non-essential amino acids,

which are the building blocks of protein. Available in capsules and powder form.

ANTIOXIDANT FORMULAS
Available from the following companies:

MegaFood
ANTIOXIDANT DAILYFOODS® Vitamin, Mineral & Herbal Formula
Contains vitamins A, C and E, zinc and selenium. DAILYFOODS® FoodState® nutrients are 100% Whole FOOD and can be taken at any time throughout the day, even on an empty stomach. Available in tablet form.

Solstice
Super Charged Anti-Oxidant
Contains vitamin E, L-glutathione, magnesium (chelate), coenzyme Q10, and other ingredients. Available in tablet form.

ASTRAGALUS EXTRACT

Planetary Formulas®
1-800-815-2333
www.sourcenaturals.com
Full Spectrum™ Astragalus Extract
Each two tablet serving combines 500 mg of standardized astragalus root extract with 500 mg of whole high grade astragalus root.

BEE PRODUCTS
Available from the following companies:

Bio-Nutritional Products
1-800-431-2582
Zell Oxygen
Contains 300 mg of fresh royal jelly, 18 amino acids, active enzymes and soluble protein. Available in glass vials.

CC Pollen
1-800-875-0096
24-Hour Royal Jelly
Available in 1 gram capsules

High Desert Bee Pollen
Available in 1 pound cans

Source Naturals®
Royal Jelly
Each capsule contains freeze-dried royal jelly equivalent to 500 mg of fresh royal jelly, in a base of rice powder.

BETA GLUCAN

Source Naturals®
A unique polysaccharide that can stimulate several aspects of immune function, such as phagocytosis and interleukin production. Each capsule contains 7.5 mg of highly purified beta-1,3-glucan, derived from baker's yeast cell wall.

BONE AND CONNECTIVE TISSUE ENHANCEMENT
Available from the following companies:

MegaFood
BONE DAILYFOODS®
Vitamin and mineral formula that provides all the essential skeletal nutrients as found in complex foods. Contains vitamins C, D3, K1, calcium, magnesium, manganese, silicon, and boron. DAILYFOODS® FoodState® nutrients are 100% Whole FOOD and can be taken at any time throughout the day, even on an empty stomach. Available in tablet form.

Source Naturals®
OPC-85™
A potent natural antioxidant derived from the bark of the European coastal pine (*Pinus maritima*) that helps to maintain the integrity of collagen and elastin, two important constituents of connective tissue. Available in 50 mg and 100 mg tablets.

Bone Balance™
Contains a 1-1 ratio of calcium and magnesium along with other bone minerals

and soy isoflavones, to provide bone support. Available in tablet form.

Recommended Reading on Bone Enhancement:
The Osteoporosis Solution by Carl Germano, R.D., C.N.S., L.D.N. (Kensington)

Broccoli Sprouts

Source Naturals®
Each tablet contains 120 mg broccoli sprouts standardized extract, yielding 150 mcg of sulforaphane.

Bromelain
Available from the following companies:

Jarrow Formulas™
Bromelain 1000
Each tablet contains 500 mg of bromelain (2000 GDU per g) providing 1000 GDU (Gelatin Digesting Units) per tablet or 1667 MCU (Milk Clotting Units).

Source Naturals®
Bromelain
Each tablet contains 500 mg of bromelain (2,000 GDU per g).

Calcium D-Glucarate
Available from the following companies:

Source Naturals®
Calcium D-Glucarate
Cellular detoxifier. Each tablet contains 500 mg of calcium D-glucarate.

Tyler, Inc.
Calcium D-Glucarate™
Available in 500 mg capsules.

Cernitin (Flower Pollen Extract)
Available from the following companies:

Cernitin America
1-800-831-9505
www.cernitinamerica.com
Clinical research documents the bene-

fits of Cernitin in promoting healthy prostate function. European studies have been conducted using Cernilton for prostate conditions.

Cernilton
Each tablet contains 60 mg of Cernitin T60 water-soluble pollen extract concentrate and 3 mg of Cernitin GBX fat-soluble pollen extract concentrate.

Cerniton T.S.—Triple Strength
Each vegi- capsule contains 180 mg of Cernitin T60 water-soluble pollen extract concentrate and 9 mg of Cernitin GBX fat-soluble pollen extract concentrate.

Graminex
1-877-472-6469
www.graminex.com
Cerniton®
Anticongestive supplement. Standardized, allergen-free, whole extract of selected pollen. Reduces prostatic volume and residual urine volume. Improves voiding difficulties. Clinical effectiveness, scientifically documented by many long-term clinical studies. Four tablets contain 250 mg of pollen extract.

Coenzyme Q10
Available from the following companies:

Carlson® Laboratories
Co-Q10
Available in 10 mg, 30 mg, 50 mg and 100 mg soft gels.

Jarrow Formulas
Co-Q10
Available in 10 mg, 30 mg, 60 mg and 100 mg capsules.

Source Naturals®
Coenzyme Q10
Available in 30 mg and100 mg softgels.

Tishcon Corporation (raw goods supplier)
516-333-3050
www.tishcon.com/ www.Q-Gel.com
This is Lee Heiman's primary CoQ10. Hydrosoluble and high bioavailability. Comes in softsules® (soft gels).

Q-Gel®: 15 mg
Q-Gel® Forte: 30 mg
Q-Gel® Plus: with 50 mg alpha lipoic acid and 100 IU natural vitamin E
Q-Gel® Ultra: 60 mg
Carni-Q-Gel®: with 30 mg CoQ10 and 250 mg L-carnitine

Tishcon's CoQ10 products are available from the following companies:

Bio Energy Nutrients (a division of Whole Foods): 1-800-627-7775
Physiologics (a division of Whole Foods): 1-800-765-6775
CountryLife: 631-231-1031
Solanova: 1-800-200-0456
Phytotherapy: 201-891-1104
Nutrimedika: 1-800-688-7462
Swanson: 1-800-437-4148
Jordets: 1-888-816-7676
Epic: 1-800-848-8442
Optimum Health: 1-800-228-1507
Doctor's Preferred: 1-800-304-1708

COLLOIDAL SILVER

Galaxy Worldwide, Inc.
1-877-968-2375
www.galaxyworldwide.com
Anti-microbial agent that was researched at the Department of Microbiology at Brigham Young University.

CLA—CONJUGATED LINOLEIC ACID

The Apothecary
Each soft gel contains 350 mg of CLA.

DIGESTIVE ENZYMES

Prevail®
Vitase® Digestive Formula
A combination of enzymes for digestive efficiency. Two capsules contain 352 mg of Pure Plant Enzymes™.

DIINDOLYMETHANE (DIM)

Tyler, Inc.
Indoplex™
Each four-capsule serving contains 22 IU of vitamin E and 60 mg of DIM. This is the first and only stable, bioavailable form of DIM, the most active and important of dietary indoles. Indoles from cruciferous vegetables have been shown to significantly influence estrogen metabolic rations. It would take more than two kilos of raw broccoli to equal the protection of four Indoplex™ capsules.

ECHINACEA

Gaia Herbs
Standardized 45 mg extract with 4% phenolic compounds and 1% isobutlyamides
Standardized 90 mg extract with 4% phenolic compounds and 1% isobutlyamides
In liquid phyto-caps, a revolutionary new delivery system for liquid herbal extracts. All phyto-caps are vegetable-based and alcohol-free.

ENZYMES WITH ENTERIC COATING
Enteric coating allows the enzyme formulation to pass through the stomach and dissolve in the lower intestine. To be used as an anti-inflammatory. Take on an empty stomach. Available from the following companies:

T.A.D. Corp.
1-800-326-0256
Poly-Zym 021
Poly-Zym 022

Priority One Health & Nutrition, L.L.C.
1-800-443-2039
Protozyme
Priority Zyme

FERMENTED SOY DRINK

EcoNugenics®
EcoGen® Fermented Soy Drink
For prostate health. When tested in a human clinical trial, slowed the PSA doubling time in a way that was not achieved by an ordinary isoflavone concentrate. Each 8 oz. amber bottle contains 150 mg of the following soy isoflavones (minimum 85% free-form): 70% Genisteins, 23% Daidzeins, and 7% Glyciteins.

FISH OILS

Available from the following companies:

Carlson® Laboratories
Norwegian Cod Liver Oil
Bottled in liquid form. High in essential fatty acids and vitamin E. Available in natural and lemon-flavored. Lee tries to take a tablespoon a day or mixes it into grains.

Norwegian Salmon Oil
Each soft gel contains 1000 mg of salmon oil. Two softgels provide 710 mg of total omega-3 fatty acids, including EPA (Eicosapentaenoic Acid), DHA (Docosahexaenoic Acid), DPA (Docosapentaenoic Acid) and ALA (Alpha-Liolenic Acid).

Super-DHA™
Each soft gel contains 1000 mg of a special blend of fish body oils, including menhaden and sardines, which are high in DHA (Docosahexaenoic Acid) and EPA (Eicosapentaenoic Acid).

Super Omega-3 Fish Oils
Contains a special concentrate of fish body oils from deep, cold-water fish, including mackerel and sardines, which are especially rich in EPA and DHA. Each soft gel provides 570 mg of total omega-3 fatty acids consisting of EPA (Eicosapentaenoic Acid), DHA (Docosahexaenoic Acid), and ALA (Alpha-Liolenic Acid).

Prevail Corporation
Eskimo-3®
Natural stable fish oil with vitamin E. Each serving of three soft gels contains 500 mg of omega-3, 240 mg of EPA, 160 mg of DHA, and 6.7 IU of vitamin E.

FLAXSEED OIL

Available from the following companies:

Matol
Omega 3-6-9
A rich source of omega 3, omega 6 and omega 9 essential fatty acids. Made from organic flaxseed—a major source of omega 3—enriched with GLA (gamma linolenic acid), high in dietary lignans and carotenoids. Available in liquid form.

Tree of Life®
High Lignan Flax Oil
Contains all the antioxidants of their original Organic Flax Oil plus the added benefits of high fiber lignans. Bottled in liquid form. Available in health food stores.

GARLIC

Wakunaga of America
Kyolic® Aged Garlic Extract (AGE)
The most scientifically researched garlic product in the world (over 220 studies), especially as it pertains to prostate and breast cancer. Research conducted at Memorial Sloan Kettering Cancer Center has verified that the compounds in Kyolic Aged Garlic Extract confirm its anti-carcinogenic properties.

Glutathione

Available from the following companies:

Carlson® Laboratories

Glutathlone Booster™
Provides the body with the nutrients needed to elevate or maintain healthy glutathione and glutathione peroxidase levels. Each capsule contains vitamins C and E, riboflavin (vitamin B-2), selenium, N-acetyl cysteine, milk thistle extract (silymarin), garlic, alpha lipoic, L-glutamine, L-glycine, asparagus concentrate, and glutathione.

Prevail Corporation

GSH Cell Support
Contains reduced L-glutathione and anthocyanidins in capsule form.

Source Naturals®

L-Glutathione
Available in 50 mg tablets

Chem-Defense™
Molybdenum/ glutathione complex. Helps to remove toxins from the body. Each orange-flavored tablet contains 1.6 mg of riboflavin (as 2.25 mg flavin mononucleotide [Coenzymated™]), 120 mcg of molybdenum (as molybdenum aspartate citrate) and 50 mg of glutathione. Taken sublingually (under the tongue) for direct absorption into the bloodstream.

Tyler, Inc.

Recancostat® 400
Each capsule contains 400 mg of reduced L-glutathione along with beet root, black currant, bilberry, elderberry, L-cysteine, and other ingredients.

Grape Seed Extract

Carlson® Laboratories

Each tablet contains 130 mg of grape seed extract and 50 mg of citrus flavonoids.

Green Tea Extract

Source Naturals®

Green Tea Extract
Each tablet contains 100 mg of standardized, patented Polyphenon 60™ green tea extract, providing at least 65 mg of polyphenols.

Indole-3-Carbinol

Life Extension
1-800-544-4440
www.lef.org
Available in 200 mg capsules.

Internal Cleansing Program

Gaia Herbs, Inc.

Supreme Cleanse™ Internal Cleansing Program
Contains certified organic and ecologically wildcrafted herbs that are specifically selected and formulated to work synergistically within the body to clear accumulated toxins and wastes.

Ipriflavone

Available from the following companies:

Jarrow Formulas

Ipriflavone 200
Supports bone health. Each capsule contains 200 mg of pharmaceutical grade ipriflavone (7-isopropoxyflavone).

Natural Balance, Inc.

Ipriflavone
Each capsule contains 200 mg of Ostivone™ brand ipriflavone.

Iprical™
Three tablets contain 600 mg of Ostivone™ ipriflavone, plus 1,000 mg of calcium and vitamin D.

Iprical Plus™
Six tablets contain 600 mg of Ostivone™ ipriflavone plus vitamins D and K, manganese, and other important minerals.

Source Naturals®
Ostivone™

Each tablet contains 300 mg of ipriflavone (Ostivone™) an isoflavone that helps maintain bone mineral density when combined with calcium.

KAVA KAVA

Source Naturals®
Kava-77™

For relaxation. Each softgel contains 140 mg of kava kava root extract (*piper methysticum*) standardized to 55% kavalactones, yielding 75 mg of kavalactones.

Gaia Herbs
Kava Kava Liquid Phyto-Cap

Contains 136 mg extract, delivering 75 kavalactones per phyto-cap, a revolutionary new delivery system for liquid herbal extracts. All phyto-caps are vegetable-based and alcohol-free.

LARIX

Larex® (raw materials supplier)
1-800-386-5300
www.larex.com

From the larch tree and the laboratory, this extract is known as *arabinogalactan*. When taken by mouth, it increases NK cell activity and induces an increased release of gamma-interferon, alpha-tumor necrosis factor, IL-1, and II-6. It is also a powerful biological response modifier. Contact Larex for a list of companies that market this product.

L-GLUTAMINE

Jarrow Formulas
Available in capsules, tablets and powder.

LIVER SUPPORT
Available from the following companies:

Prevail®
Metabolic Liver Formula™

Contains 80% silymarin with Plant Enzymes™, black radish root, dandelion root, beet leaf, kelp and other effective ingredients.

Solstice
Liver Formula

Aids in the rebuilding of the body's ability to process necessary nutrients and eliminate toxins. Contains beta carotene, vitamins B-1, B-2, B-6, B-12, niacinamide, magnesium citrate, desiccated liver, silymarin, taraxicum, cardus marianus, yarrow, and beet leaf. Available in tablet form.

Source Naturals®
Liver Guard™

Contains lipoic acid, silymarin and N-acetyl cysteine (NAC) to support healthy liver function. Also contains herbs for cleansing the liver as well as choline and inositol for preventing fat from depositing in the liver. Available in tablets.

LYCOPENE
Available from the following companies:

Healthy Origins
1-888-228-6650
Lyc-O-mato

This is a more powerful lycopene developed in Israel. Available in 15 mg soft gels.

Jarrow Formulas™
Lyco-Sorb™

A natural GMO-free tomato source of lycopene in a high absorption format. Each softgel contains 10 mg of lycopene and 4 mg of gamma tocopherol.

MELATONIN
Available from the following companies:

Jarrow Formulas
Melatonin Sustain™

Sustained release melatonin. Each tablet contains 1 mg melatonin, 2 mg vitamin B6 (Pyridoxine HCl) and 100 mg magnesium (from oxide).

Source Naturals®

Melatonin
Available in 1 mg, 3 mg and 5 mg tablets.

Melatonin
Sublingual. Available in 1 mg, 2.5 mg and 5 mg orange or peppermint flavored tablets that are taken sublingually (under the tongue) for direct absorption into the bloodstream.

MODIFIED CITRUS PECTIN
Available from the following companies:

EcoNugenics®
PectaSol® Modified Citrus Pectin
For prostate health. Clinically proven to considerably slow the PSA doubling time in prostate cancer patients. Also enhances immune function. Available in powder form—454 g per bottle—and capsules—800 mg per capsule.

Source Naturals®
Modified Citrus Pectin
Available in powder form. Two level teaspoons contain approximately 5 g of modified citrus pectin.

MOLYBDENUM

Source Naturals®
Chem-Defense™
Molybdenum/ glutathione complex. Helps to remove toxins from the body. Each orange-flavored tablet contains 1.6 mg of riboflavin (as 2.25 mg flavin mononucleotide [Coenzymated™]), 120 mcg of molybdenum (as molybdenum aspartate citrate) and 50 mg of glutathione. Taken sublingually (under the tongue) for direct absorption into the bloodstream.

MSM
Available from the following companies:

Carlson®
MSM Sulfur
Each capsule contains 1,000 mg of MSM (methylsulfonylmethane), providing 334 mg of organic dietary sulfur.

Jarrow Formulas
MSM
Available in 750 mg and 100 mg capsules and 200 g and 454 g powder.

Natural Balance
MSM
Available in tablets and powder

MULTIVITAMIN AND MINERAL FORMULATIONS
Available from the following companies:

MegaFood
LIFESTYLE™ DAILYFOODS® Vitamin, Mineral & Herbal Formula
This unique formulation delivers nutrients in the FoodState® for maximum utilization. Recent scientific studies have proven that nutrients function at their peak when consumed as they naturally occur in food. Because MegaFood's formulas are food, they are particularly effective. DAILYFOODS® FoodState® nutrients are 100% Whole FOOD and can be taken at any time throughout the day, even on an empty stomach. Available in tablet form.

The Synergy Company™
Vita Synergy™ for Men
1-800-723-0277
Another fine, all-inclusive vitamin-mineral-botanical supplement made from 100% natural whole food, no binders or fillers.

Mushrooms
Available from the following companies:

EcoNugenics®

MycoCeutics®

Balanced ratio of ten immune-enhancing mushrooms: *reishi, maitake, shitake, hericum, cordydeps, coriolus, umbellatus (polyporus), wood ear, poria,* and *tremella.* Grown on a bed of organic brown rice with additional Beta-1,3-glucan added to enhance the immune-boosting Beta-glucans (Beta-1,3 and Beta-1,6) naturally occurring in the mushrooms. Available in 600 mg BSE-free gelatin capsules.

Maitake Products, Inc.

1-800-747-7418

www.maitake.com

Maitake D-fraction® Extract

Studies in Japan and elsewhere indicate that this product may be effective against cancer. Every six drops contains a minimum of pure and active 6.6 mg of beta-glucan in a standardized extract.

Mai Green™ Tea

Contains organically grown maitake mushroom and premier Japanese green tea (matcha) leaves. Low in caffeine. Available in tea bags.

N-Acetyl Cysteine

N-acetyl cysteine is an amino acid that is valuable for the production of glutathione in our bodies. Available from the following companies:

Carlson® Laboratories

N-A-C

Available in 500 mg capsules and 100 g powder.

Source Naturals®

N-Acetyl Cysteine

Available in 600 mg and 1,000 mg tablets.

Niacin

Tyler, Inc.

Niacinol™

One capsule provides 500 mg of niacin.

Natural Killer Cell Support

Solstice

NK Support

Contains arabinogalactan, 24 essential amino acids and acid enzymes. Available in powdered form. Mix with juice or water.

PC SPES

Available from the following companies:

BotanicLab™

1-800-242-5555

www.botaniclab.com

BotanicLab™ is the primary distributor of PC SPES, which has had encouraging results in clinical trials involving prostate cancer patients at well-respected university research centers, including UCSF Medical Center, Columbia-Presbyterian Medical Center, the Cancer Institute of New Jersey, and the University of Kentucky. In addition, several *in vivo* and *in vitro* studies have been conducted at various well-known research laboratories and published in medical journals. For information about PC SPES, contact BotanicLab™ through their toll-free phone number or visit them on their website.

Two other highly recommended organizations that sell PC SPES:

The Apothecary

N.E.E.D.S.

Plant Sterols and Sterolins

Moducare Sterinol™

Moducare Sterinol is a patented blend of plant sterols and sterolins that possess a powerful anti-cancer effect. Plant sterols and sterolins have been used for over twenty years by German urologists for the treatment of enlarged prostate and prostate cancer. It has been shown to rapidly lower PSA, increase natural killer cell activity, halt the conversion of testosterone and reduce inflammation and edema. Moducare, researched by Professor Patrick Bouic, is used to normalize or balance immune function for the treatment of cancer, autoimmune disease, allergies and other immune-mediated diseases. Thousands of research studies have been published worldwide on plant sterols and sterolins including140 double-blind trials in humans. See *The Immune System Cure* published by Kensington for complete documentation on plant sterols and sterolins.

Available from the following companies:

Moducare Sterinol
1-877-297-7332
www.moducare.com

Natural Balance
1-800-833-8737
www.naturalbalance.com
(In Canada) Purity Life Health Products
1-800-265-2615

POTASSIUM
Available from the following companies:

Carlson® Laboratories
Potassium
Each table provides 99 mg of potassium from 595 mg of potassium gluconate

Matol
KM®
A very potent and effective compound. Liquid extract for maximum absorption.

Each serving of two tablespoons contains 562 mg of potassium and 14 herbs, which provide powerful essential minerals. Also available in capsules.

PROBIOTICS (ACIDOPHILUS)
Available from the following companies:

Bio-K + Plus International, Inc.
1-800-593-2465
Bio-K + Plus®
High concentration of active acidophilus CL285 and casei—a minimum of 50 billion per 3.5 oz. Comes in an edible cream-like form that must be refrigerated. Available from your local health-food store or contact Bio-K + Plus for where you can purchase this product.

Jarrow Formulas™
Jarro-Dophilus™
High potency, non-dairy, multi-strain probiotic. Each 280 mg capsule contains six species of the hardiest of the lactobacilli and bifidobacteria at a potency of 10-15 billion per gram.
Jarro-Dophilus™ + FOS (available in capsules and powder)
Jarro-Dophilus™ + Colostrum (capsules)
Jarro-Dophilus™ + Lactoferrin (capsules)

Prevail®
Inner Ecology™
Intestinal balancing acidophilus formula. Dairy-free. Contains specially prepared *lactobacillus* and *bifidobacteria*. Available in powder form.

PROSTATE SUPPORT

Source Naturals®
Prosta Response—Prostate Support
Promotes healthy prostate function. Each tablet contains soy phytoestrogen extract (non-GMO soy, providing 31 mg naturally occurring isoflavones consisting of genistein, daidzen, and glycitein),

quercetin, alanine, glycine, glutamic acid, nettle extract (16:1), pumpkin seed oil extract (25% fatty acids), pygeum Africanum 30:1 Ext. (standardized to 2.5% sterols), green tea extract (standardized for min. 95% total polyphenols), lycopene (standardized to 5%), vitamin D3, vitamin E, zinc (monomethione) selenium (sodium selenite and L-selenomethione), and other healthful ingredients.

PULSATILLA

See page 261 at the end of the Resource Section for more information.

PYCNOGENOL

Source Naturals®
Pycnogenol®
Proanthocyanidin Complex. Available in 25 mg, 50 mg, 75 mg and 100 mg tablets.

Pycnogenol® Complex
Antioxidant Formula. Combines pycnogenol and proanthodyn (grape seed extract), antioxidants and plantioxidants (plant-derived antioxidants. Available in tablet form.

QUERCETIN
Available from the following companies:

Jarrow Formulas
Quercetin 500™
Bioflavonoid antioxidant available in 500 mg capsules.

Source Naturals®

Activated Quercetin™
Nonallergenic bioflavonoid complex. Three tablets contain 1,000 mg quercetin, 600 mg vitamin C (magnesium ascorbate), 47 mg magnesium (magnesium ascorbate), and 300 mg bromelain (2,000 GDU per g).

NutraSpray™ Quercetin
Seasonal bioflavonoid complex. Each spray contains 50 mg quercetin. Natural tangerine flavor.

RED CLOVER

Gaia Herbs, Inc.
Red Clover Supreme
The herbs in this compound are classic blood and lymphatic alteratives which alter the catabolic tissue conditions and bring about an improved state of well-being through improved metabolism and elimination. Available in liquid extract form.

RESPIRATORY INFECTIONS

Matol
Biomune OSF™ Express Nasal Spray
Homeopathic medicine conatining Ai/E10. Can be helpful for treating symptoms of upper respiratory infections, which can weaken the immune system. This product can be used as a complement to the dietary supplement, Biomune OSF™ Plus (listed under AIDBCWE).

ST. JOHN'S WORT

Gaia Herbs
Standardized 0.5 hypericins 90 mg extract
Standardized double strength 0.5 hypericins 90 mg extract
In liquid phyto-caps, a revolutionary new delivery system for liquid herbal extracts. All phyto-caps are vegetable-based and alcohol-free.

SAM-e

Jarrow Formulas
SAM-e 200
(S-Adenosyl Methionine)
Each enteric coated tablet contains 200 mg elemental from 400 mg of SAM-e tosylate disulfate.

SELENIUM

Available from the following companies:

Carlson® Laboratories

Selenium
Yeast-free. Each capsule contains organically bound selenium from L-selenomethionine, providing 200 mcg of selenium.

E-Sel
Natural-source vitamin E and organic selenium. Two soft gels contain 400 IU of vitamin E (d-alpha tocopheryl acetate derived from soybean oil) and 100 mcg of selenium (from L-selenomethione).

Cypress

559-229-7850
www.cypsystems.com
SelenoExcell™ High Selenium Yeast
This product was used in the Nutritional Prevention of Cancer Study conducted by the University of Arizona by Larry C. Clark, M.P.H., Ph.D. Contact Cypress for the various supplement companies that carry this product.

Source Naturals®

Selenomax®
Contains selenium from Selenomax® high selenium yeast. Available in 100 mcg and 200 mcg tablets.

SHARK LIVER OIL

Scandinavian Laboratories

570-897-7735
Oceana®
Each soft gel contains 570 mg of purified whole shark liver oil from North Sea deep water sharks, naturally combining 110 mg of squalene with 325 mg of diacylglycerol ethers (D.A.G.E.) and 125 mg of alkylglycerols. Also contains some omega-3 fatty acids. Infants fortunate to be breast-fed, get these ingredients from their mothers' milk.

SOY PRODUCTS

Available from the following companies:

Carlson® Laboratories

Easy Soy® Gold
Each tablet contains 325 mg of high isoflavone concentrate, providing 130 mg of soy isoflavones, including 60 mg of genistein and genistin, 58 mg of daidzein and daidzin, and 12 mg of glycitein and glycitin.

EcoNugenics®

EcoGen® Soybean Isoflavone Concentrate
A unique, potent source of isoflavones. Contains significant quantities of genistein, daidzein, and glycetein. Available in powder form (1 tsp = 2 g) and 750 mg tablets.

S.O.D. (SUPER OXIDE DISMUTASE)

Nutratech, Inc. (raw goods manufacturer)

973-882-7773
www.nutratechinc.com
Bioavailable S.O.D. in a completely vegan formulation. Contact Nutratech for a list of companies that market this product.

THYMUS GLAND SUPPORT

EcoNugenics®

TLC Thymic Longevity Compound
The active ingredient is the essential thymus-produced protein that sets up a virtual cascade of immune stimulation, beginning with T-4 lymphocytes. Each single dose 4 mcg packet contains 12 trillion biologically active molecules of protein in a base of about 1 gram of malto-dextrin powder. Take under the tongue on an empty stomach.

TURMERIC EXTRACT

Source Naturals®
Each tablet contains 350 mg of turmeric, yielding 95% curcumin, and 50 mg of bromelain (pineapple enzyme) (2,000 GDU per gram).

VITAMINS A & D
Available from the following companies:

Carlson® Laboratories
Vitamins A and D3
Each soft gel contains 10,000 IU of natural source vitamin A and 400 IU of natural source vitamin D3 from fish liver oil.

Solstice
P-Care™
Balanced source of vitamins A and D and an excellent source of CoQ10 and niacin. Available in tablet form.

Source Naturals®
Vitamins A and D
Each tablet contains 10,000 IU of vitamin A and 400 IU of vitamin D.

VITAMIN B COMPLEX
Available from the following companies:

Carlson® Laboratories
B-Compleet™
Provides all the B-vitamins plus vitamin C in a balanced formulation. Available in tablets.

Source Naturals®
Coenzymate™ B Complex
Contains coenzymes along with a full range of B-vitamins and CoQ10. Available in orange or peppermint flavored tablets that are taken sublingually (under the tongue) for direct absorption into the bloodstream.

VITAMIN C
Available from the following companies:

Carlson® Laboratories
Mild-C Chewable
Buffered form of chewable vitamin C that is non-acidic and gentle to the teeth. Each orange and tangerine flavored tablet supplies 250 mg of vitamin C and 28 mg of calcium.

MegaFood
Complex C
Vitamin C as found in food, is a very complex nutrient of which ascorbic acid is only one factor. Complex C DAILY-FOODS® contains all the food factors, such as bioflavonoids, that occur in food and enhance its effectiveness. DAILY-FOODS® FoodState® nutrients are 100% Whole FOOD and can be taken at any time throughout the day, even on an empty stomach. Available in 250 mg tablets.

Source Naturals®
C-500
Each tablet provides 500 mg of vitamin C (ascorbic acid) and 50 mg of rose hips.

C-1000 Timed Release
Provides a gradual release over a prolonged period of time. Each tablet provides 1,000 mg of vitamin C (ascorbic acid) and 100 mg of rose hips.

Wellness C-1000™
Each tablet contains 1,000 mg of vitamin C and several sources of bioflavonoids and alpha-lipoic acid.

VITAMIN D
Available from the following companies:

Biotics Research Corporation
1-800-231-5777
www.bioticsresearch.com
Vitamin D

An oil in water emulsion in which vitamin D has been dispersed. Each drop supplies 400 IU of emulsified vitamin D.

Carlson®
Vitamin D3
Natural source vitamin D3 from fish liver oil. Available in 400 IU and 1,000 IU soft gels.

VITAMIN E
Available from the following companies:

Carlson® Laboratories

d-Alpha Gems™
Each tiny soft gel contains 400 IU of vitamin E (d-alpha tocopherol acetate).

E-Gems® Plus
Each soft gel contains vitamin E derived from soybean oil, supplying alpha-tocopherol plus mixed tocopherols. Available in three strengths: 200 IU, 400 IU and 800 IU.

Jarrow Formulas
Oil E
Vitamin E as 100% natural form d-alpha tocopherol with mixed tocopherols. Available in 400 IU and 600 IU soft gels.

MegaFood
E & Selenium DAILYFOODS®
In foods, vitamin E and selenium are always found together. Vitamin E doesn't work without the presence of selenium and vice versa. This combination offers these two important nutrients as they naturally occur in food, and therefore provides maximum protection. DAILY-FOODS® FoodState® nutrients are 100% Whole FOOD and can be taken at any time throughout the day, even on an empty stomach. Each tablet contains 100 IU of vitamin E and 100 mg of selenium.

Source Naturals®

Vitamin E
Each softgel contains 400 IU of natural vitamin E (d-alpha tocopherol) and 67 mg of mixed tocopherols (d-beta, d-gamma, and d-delta). In a base of soybean oil.

Tocotrienol Antioxidant Complex™
Each softgel contains a total of 34 mg of tocotrienols (29.8 mg gamma-tocotrienol, 3 mg alpha-tocotrienol, and 1.3 mg delta-tocotrienol) and 100 IU of vitamin E (d-alpha tocopherol)

WHEY PROTEIN
Available from the following companies:

Jarrow Formulas™
American Whey Protein
High in glutamine and specially ultrafiltered to be low in lactose, fat, and carbohydrates. Available in powdered form in vanilla creme, Caribbean chocolate and unflavored.

Metagenics
1-800-692-9400
Bio Pure Protein
Available in powdered form. Pure whey protein with natural immunoglobulins.

Wellsprings
619-469-8196
www.immunepro.com
ImmunePro™
Research has proven that ingesting undenatured whey protein concentrate can boost an individual's albumin levels and substantially increase the production of glutathione. Glutathione has been clinically proven to play a major role in eliminating many carcinogens and in maintaining a vital immune system for anti-tumor defense. Available in powdered form.

ZINC

Available from the following companies:

Carlson® Laboratories
Zinc
Contains zinc from zinc gluconate in 15 mg and 50 mg tablets.

Jarrow Formulas™
Zinc Balance 15™
A synergistic combination of OptiZinc™

brand zinc monomethionate and copper gluconate in a 15:1 zinc/copper ratio. Each capsule contains 15 mg of zinc (as monomethionine) and 1 mg of copper (as gluconate).

Source Naturals®
OptiZinc®
Each tablet contains 30 mg of zinc (from 150 mg of OptiZinc® zinc monomethionine) and 300 mcg of copper (sebacate).

Special Resource Section (including foods, teas, juices, etc.)

ANTI-AGING

American Academy of Anti-Aging Medicine
773-528-4833
www.worldhealth.net

Keeping alive is obviously the most important thing that a cancer patient can do. The American Academy of Anti-Aging Medicine (AAM) is a wonderful organization dedicated to increasing both the quality and length of the human life-span. This organization is a society of 8,500 physicians from 55 countries around the world, which provides reliable medical education and information to the general public on the latest breakthroughs in medicine, science, and technology.

BEET JUICE CRYSTALS

Bio-Nutritional Products
1-800-431-2582
Excellent for prostate health. Dr. Stoff recommends using beets regularly. This product contains many nutrients. Mix with water for a tasty and nutritious drink.

BOTTLED WATER

Mountain Valley Water
1-800-643-1501
A fine, slightly alkaline water, bottled in glass from a pure, natural spring. In Lee

Heiman's opinion, this is the best bottled in glass water available.

FLAX

Health From The Sun
1-800-447-2229
FiPro FLAX™
Organic ground flaxseeds combined with fermented soy meal and other ingredients. Crunchy texture and delicious, nutty taste. Sprinkle on salads, cereal, soup and pasta. Available in healthfood stores.

GRAINS

Available from the following companies:

INF—InterNatural Foods
201-909-0808
McCann's Steelcut Wholegrain Irish Oatmeal
High in B vitamins, calcium, protein and fiber, while low in fat with no added salt.

Lundberg Family Farms
530-882-4550 (ext. 319)
www.lundberg.com
Grower and marketer of organic rice and rice products. This is my favorite rice company. They have an amazing variety of rices, rice cakes, etc. Reliable quality.

POWDERED GREEN DRINKS

Available from the following companies:

The Synergy Company™
Pure Synergy™
Certified organic superfood formula that is a blend of more than sixty of nature's finest and most potent superfoods, including 11 ocean and fresh water algae, 7 grass juices, 17 Chinese and 10 Western herbs, 5 immune-supporting Asian mushrooms, plant enzymes, natural lecithin, royal jelly and natural antioxidants.

Wakunaga
Kyo-Green®
A combination of organically grown barley and wheat grasses, kelp, chlorella and brown rice. Two teaspoons provide the nutrients of a serving of deep green leafy vegetables.

JUICER

Miracle Exclusives, Inc.
1-800-645-6360
www.miracleexclusives.com
Stainless Steel Juice Extractor, Model MJ 7000-1
This is a relatively small machine (only 14" high) that is very effective and easy to clean. Miracle Exclusives has a full line of juicers and a soy milk-making machine.

NONI

Tahiti Traders
1-800-842-5309
www.tahititraders.com
Tahiti Trader's Noni Juice
Try making this good tasting nutritional drink a part of your diet by drinking one "shot" (2 ounces) of concentrated noni juice daily. This juice acts as a tremendous aid for digestion and it appears to help all body organs. It is also a great analgesic. Tahiti Trader's noni juice has an extremely high concentration of noni fruit per ounce.

ORGANIC TEAS

The Republic of Tea
1-800-354-5530
www.republicoftea.com
Growers and marketers of certified organic teas, including green teas and herbal teas. Available in bulk or in tea bags at natural food stores, gourmet and specialty food stores, and select department stores, cafés and restaurants.

POULTRY

Sheltons Poultry, Inc.
1-800-541-1833
Free-range chicken and turkey and no added antibiotics. Available in natural foods stores.

PURIFIED WATER

Merlin Water
1-800-982-2890
www.merlinwater.com
This is the special, doubled-purified water that Lee described in his personal case history.

SEAFOOD
Available from the following companies:

Capilano Pacific
1-877-391-WILD (9453)
www.capilanopacific.com
Wildfish™
This company is a wonderful source for wild-caught salmon. Most of the salmon available in restaurants and stores are farm-raised. Usually this means medications such as antibiotics have been added to the feed, as well as synthetic coloring. Wild-caught salmon has none of these problems and a high level of omega-3 fatty acids and much less fat than farm-raised salmon. It tastes better as well. Also available: halibut, tuna and lox without any added chemicals.

New World Marketing Group
203-221-8008
Sardines
Packed in pure virgin olive oil and virgin olive oil with garlic. Very high in omega-3 fatty acids. They also have water-packed sardines which contain less sodium. Available in natural foods stores.

Seafood Direct
1-800-732-1836
Salmon caught in the wild, including Wild Alaskan Salmon, King Salmon and Sockeye Salmon. Available in frozen filets and steaks. Also available in jars and cans.

SELECTED HERBAL VEGETABLE SOUP MIXTURE

Sun Farm Corporation
203-777-6639
www.sunfarmcorp.com
Freeze-dried soup with many ingredients that contain immune-enhancing components.

Stevia
Wisdom of the Ancients®
1-800-899-9908
www.wisdomherbs.com
Natural sweetener made from whole leaf Stevia (S*tevia rebaudiana Bertoni*) 6:1 concentrated extract. Available in concentrated tablets, liquid, and as a tea.

TREE OF LIFE®
www.treeoflife.com

There are many fine healthfood stores all over the country that carry top-notch products. Many stores are supplied by an excellent company known as Tree of Life, a distributor of high quality natural foods at moderate prices. When shopping at healthfood stores, you can ask for Tree of Life products. If a store doesn't carry a particular product, they can order it for you.

Tree of Life Frozen Organic Vegetables
Lee always stock these in his freezer because he doesn't always have access to organic vegetables:
Broccoli Cuts
Green Peas
Spinach

Tree of Life Frozen Fruit
Organic fruits are loaded with nutrients. These are often difficult to obtain:
Strawberries
Blueberries
Raspberries

Tree of Life Frozen Smoothie Makers
Fresh-frozen chunks of 100% organic fruit. Ideal for juicing.
Banana, Rasberry, Strawberry

Tree of Life Organic Tamari and Soyu
Made from organic soybeans and wheat. Excellent for steamed vegetables and fish.
Shoyu
Wheat-Free Tamari

Tree of Life Organic Extra Virgin Olive Oil

Bella Via Organic Extra Virgin Olive Oil
Made from the first pressing of 100% organic olives imported from the Andalusia region of Spain.

Avoiding Environmental Toxins

In this book, you have learned the importance of avoiding toxins in the food you eat, the water you drink, the air you breathe, and in virtually every product you use, from shampoos and toothpaste to cleaning products for your home. The companies listed here are those Lee Heiman has personally found to be of the highest quality. If you cannot find their products at your local healthfood store, please contact these companies directly for the store nearest you.

DENTAL PRODUCTS

Woodstock Natural Products, Inc.
The Natural Dentist™
1-800-615-6895
Lee's favorite toothpastes and mouth rinses, formulated by a holistic dentist, containing soothing herbs and no alcohol, sugar, or harsh chemicals. These products have been clinically proven to kill germs that cause gum disease.
Toothpaste: mint, cinnamon and fluoride-free mint
Mouth rinse: mint, cinnamon, cherry-flavored

Peelu U.S.A.
1-800-457-3358
The fibers and extracts of the Peelu tree have been used for centuries in Asia and in the Middle East for dental care. Peelu products are sugar-free, with no artificial sweeteners or preservatives, no chemicals or abrasives, and no animal testing. Peelu Dental Fibers: finely ground, easy-to-apply powder that cleans and brightens teeth. Available in peppermint, spearmint, or mint-free flavors.

Dr. Tung's Natural Dental Products
1-800-960-7144
Manufacturer of a stainless steel tongue cleaner that helps to prevent plaque and reduce bad breath.

REMOVAL OF MERCURY AMALGAM FILLINGS

To find a holistic dentist who can safely remove mercury fillings, contact:

International Academy of Oral Medicine and Toxicology
Michael F. Ziff, D.D.S. Executive Director
P.O. Box 60851
Orlando, FL 32860
407-298-2450
An organization of mercury-free dentists.

These are two of the finest dentists in the New York City area who can safely remove mercury amalgam fillings:

Victor Zeines, D.D.S.
212-813-9461
www.natdent.com

Robert Veligdan, D.M.D.
212-753-1119

N.E.E.D.S.
1-800-634-1380
www.needs.com
An excellent resource for top-notch environmental products, including:

AIREOX Air Purifier (Model 45)
Removes mold spores, pollen dust, formaldehyde, and more.

Elite Shower Filter and Massager: for removing chlorine, heavy metals and bacteria.

Teslar Watch
"The watch that protects" you from many unrecognized dangers of electromagnetic fields produced by cell phones, computers, televisions, telephones, automobiles, fluorescent lights, etc. By adding the Teslar chip to the watch, your Teslar not only tells time but also protects you from harmful ELF's. According to Dr. Doris Rapp, M.D., Dr. John Upledger, D.O., Dr. Valerie Hunt, Ph.D., and Dr. Scott Morley, M.D. (M.A.) "the Teslar watch performs as advertised".

HOUSEHOLD CLEANING PRODUCTS

ECover®
1-800-449-4925
www.ecover.com
Leading manufacturer of environmentally safe and toxic free household cleaning products. Their line includes dish and laundry products and a full range of household cleansers. Available in health food stores

PILLOWS
Available from the following companies:

Boxi™ Pillows
1-877-YESBOXI (937-2694)
Dual-chambered pillow that is box-shaped to deliver more filling at the edge where it supports your neck. The top chamber holds fluffed wool batting to cushion your face in comfort. The bottom holds organic buckwheat hulls that conform to your contours and hold your head, neck and spine in alignment. Available in certified organic or conventionally grown cotton casing. Comes in several sizes. Provides a very restful sleep.

KB Cotton Pillows, Inc.
1-800-544-3752
www.kcottonpillows.com
Also available from N.E.E.D.S.
100% cotton pillows to avoid foam pillows that emit formaldehyde, fire retardant and pesticides. The most comfortable regular pillow I've slept on.

NATURAL COSMETICS
Available from the following companies:

Carlson®
E-Gem® Oil Drops
Each drop contains 10 IU of vitamin E. 5000 IU of vitamin E per ½ ounce. Apply externally to aid and soften skin.

E-Gem® Organic Shampoo
Formulated with vitamin E, vitamins A and D, panthenol and protein.

Garden Fresh Soap
100% vegetarian. Contains aloe vera, avocado, cucumber, carrot oil, olive oil and other ingredients.

Jason Natural Cosmetics
1-800-JASON-05
www.jason-natural.com

Chamomile Liquid Satin Soap™ with Pump
Natural Sea Kelp Shampoo

Jason Natural carries a full line of cosmetics that are free of toxic substances, including natural underarm deodorant and alcohol-free shaving cream and after-shave lotion.

WATER FILTER
High Tech Health, Inc.
1-800-794-5355

Ionizer Plus

This is the best water filter I have ever used. It provides superior water filtration to 1/10 of a micron (below bacteria levels) and ultraviolet to eliminate viruses. The greatest benefit of this filtration system is its ability to ionize minerals in water, thereby increasing the mineral bioavailability and the PH. This is an excellent method of eliminating digestive and other problems caused by over-acidity. For me, the machine is ideal because it allows me to adjust the alkaline level of the water I drink, and maintaining an alkaline PH is important for cancer patients. If you are not completely satisfied with this product, the company will refund your money.

Dr. Stoff has designed and tested a new product, P-Kare, which contains many of the ingredients he recommends throughout this book.

P-Kare
Solstice
1-800-765-7842
Contains pulsatilla 50mg, nettle root extract 100mg, inositol-hexanicotinata 600mg, CoQ-10 50mg, L-selenomethionine 75mg, vitamin D_3 400 IU, vitamin A 2000 IU, lycopene 10mg, pygeum 100mg, beta sitosterol 10mg, pyridoxine 5 phosphate 10mg, indole 3 carbinol 30mg, gamma fraction tocotrienols 25mg, quercetin 50mg. Available in tablets.

ENVIRONMENTAL PHYSICIAN:
Dr. Sherry Rogers is a pre-eminent authority in environmental medicine who specializes in finding the environmental causative factors of disease. She is available for personal phone consultations (315-488-2856). One of her books, *Wellness Against All Odds*, is a must for all cancer patients. Get this and her other dozen books and referenced monthly subscription newsletter (free sample available) from 1-800-846-6687 or prestigepublishing.com.

Bibliography

Anderson, Greg, *The Triumphant Patient,* Thomas Nelson Pub., TN, 1992

Cooper, David, *The Heart of Stillness,* Bell Tower, New York, 1992

Cousins, Norman, *Anatomy of an Illness,* W.W. Norton & Co., New York, 1979

Cousins, Norman, *Head First: The Biology of Hope,* E.P. Dutton, New York, 1989

Cousins, Norman, *The Healing Heart,* W.W. Norton & Co., New York, 1983

Cousins, Norman, *Human Options,* W.W. Norton & Co., New York, 1981

Demet, William C., M.D., Ph.D., *The Promise of Sleep,* Random House, New York, 1999

De Salvo, Louise, Ph.D., *Writing as a Way of Healing,* Harper, San Francisco, CA, 1999

Fawcett, Ann and Smith, Cynthia, *Cancer-Free,* Japan Pub. Inc., New York, 1991

Hirshberg, Caryle and Barasch, Marc, *Remarkable Recovery,* Riverhead Books, New York, 1998

Kaufman, Barry Neil, *Happiness is a Choice,* Fawcett Columbine, New York, 1991

Labowitz, Shoni, *Miraculous Living,* Fireside, New York, 1996

Le Shan, Lawrence, Ph.D., *Cancer as a Turning Point,* Penguin Books, New York, 1994

Levine, Stephen, *Healing Into Life and Death,* Doubleday, New York, 1987

Maley, Michael, Ph.D., *Living in the Question,* Bodysmart Pub., MN, 1995

Matthews, Dale, M.D. and Clark, Connie, *The Faith Factor,* Penguin Putnam, Inc., New York 1998

Mees, L.F.C., M.D., *Blessed by Illness,* Anthroposophic Press, New York,1983

Millman, Dan, *The Path of the Peaceful Warrior,* H.J. Kramer, CA, 1984

Pennebacker, James, Ph.D., *Opening Up,* Guilford Press, VT, 1997

Pert, Candace, Ph.D., *Molecules of Emotion,* Simon & Schuster, New York,1997

Quillin, Patrick, *Beating Cancer with Nutrition,* Nutrition Times Press, CA 1998

Siegel, Bernie, *How to Live Between Office Visits,* HarperCollins, New York,1993

Siegel, Bernie, *Love, Medicine and Miracles,* Harper & Row, New York,1988

Siegel, Bernie, *Peace, Love and Healing,* Harper & Row, New York,1989

Siegel, Bernie, *Prescription for Living,* Harper Collins, New York,1998

Stoff, Jesse, M.D. and Pellegrino, Charlie, Ph.D., *Chronic Fatigue Syndrome: The Hidden Epidemic,* Harper Collins, New York,1992

Weil, Andrew, M.D., *Health and Healing,* Houghton Mifflin Co., New York,1995

Weil, Andrew, M.D., *Natural Health, Natural Medicine,* Houghton Mifflin Co., New York,1998

Weil, Andrew, M.D., *Spontaneous Healing,* Fawcett Columbine, New York,1995

Whitmont, Edward C., *The Alchemy of Healing,* North Atlantic Books, New York,1993

Williams, Wendy, *The Power Within,* W.W. Norton & Co., New York,1987

Winston, David, AHG, *Saw Palmetto for Men and Women,* Storey Books, VT 1999

Index